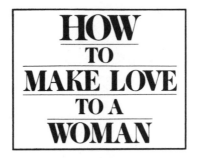

HOW
TO
MAKE LOVE
TO A
WOMAN

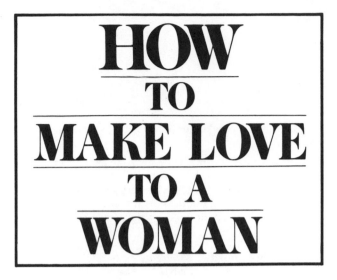

HOW TO MAKE LOVE TO A WOMAN

By
MICHAEL MORGENSTERN

with
STEVEN NAIFEH
and
GREGORY WHITE SMITH

DIADEM BOOKS
NEW YORK

For the Fair Sex

Copyright © 1982 by Michael Morgenstern

All rights reserved.

This 1986 edition is published by Diadem Books, distributed by
Crown Publishers, Inc., 225 Park Avenue South, New York, New
York 10003, by arrangement with Clarkson N. Potter, Inc.

Printed and Bound in the United States of America

Library of Congress Cataloging-in-Publication Data
Morgenstern, Michael.
    How to make love to a woman.
    1. Sex instruction for men.   2. Women—Sexual behavior.
3. Sex (Psychology)   4. Love.   I. Naifeh, Steven W., 1952-
II. Smith, Gregory White.   III. Title.
HQ36.M68   1986   613.9'6   85-27513
ISBN 0-517-60525-2

m l k

Contents

Acknowledgments

First, I want to thank the dozens of people who spoke so candidly to me in the interviews that form the basis of this book. There are too many to thank individually, but I cannot help acknowledging the contributions of a few of the most helpful: Jim Allen, Beth Atkin, Orith Bender, Norma Lee Clark, Joseph Hartzler, Susan Hunter, Karen Hutson, Melody Kimmel, Susan Korb, Alice Long, Helen Manning, Roni Margolis, Bonnie Naifeh, Wendy Resnick, Christine Reynolds, Gaby Rodgers, Arthur Slaven, Nancy Starr, Maurizia Tovo, and Dmitri Vassilopoulos. Barbara Mitchell, M.D., Department of Obstetrics and Gynecology, and Robert Wilkins, M.D., Department of Radiology, both of the Mount Sinai Medical Center of New York, provided pertinent medical information and advice. In addition, special thanks are due to Dr. Brian C. Campden-Main, a psychiatrist, and his wife, Mary Linda Sara, co-directors of the Marital Sexual Therapy Institute in Fairfax County, Virginia, and two psychologists, Dr. Lewis M. K. Long of Alexandria, Virginia, and Dr. Marilyn Machlowitz of New York. The gentlemen at Ray's Escort Service in New York also made an important contribution to the book.

ACKNOWLEDGMENTS

Lewis M. K. Long of Alexandria, Virginia, and Dr. Marilyn Machlowitz of New York. The gentlemen at Ray's Escort Service in New York also made an important contribution to the book.

My agent, Connie Clausen, was gracious and supportive throughout the writing of the book. I also want to thank the charming Carol Southern, my editor at Clarkson N. Potter, for her extraordinary assistance.

Finally, two friends, Steven Naifeh in New York and Gregory White Smith in Los Angeles, were of inestimable help in researching and writing the book. Without their contributions, the book would not have been possible.

—M.M.
New York City

"How to handle a woman?
There's a way," said a wise old man,
"A way known by every woman
Since the whole rigmarole began."

"Do I flatter her?" I begged him answer.
"Do I threaten or cajole or plead?
Do I brood or play the gay romancer?"
Said he, smiling, "No, indeed."

"How to handle a woman?
Mark me well, I will tell you, sir.
The way to handle a woman
Is to love her,
Simply love her,
Merely love her,
Love her,
Love her."

Lerner and Loewe,
"How to Handle a Woman"
from *Camelot*

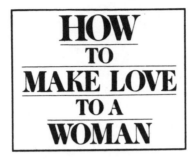

HOW
TO
MAKE LOVE
TO A
WOMAN

ONE

What Do Women Want?

L ike most men my age, I was exposed to sex long
before I was exposed to love. Most of the women I
know arrived at the same point by just the opposite
route: they fantasized about love long before they knew
about sex. To this day, I remain convinced that these
different paths help explain why men and women are so
confused about the relationship between these two great
forces: love and sex.

That, in a nutshell, is what this book is about: sex
and love. How they're different, how they're alike, and
most important, how they're inseparable. If you had
questioned every man in America, every year, over the
last two decades about the relationship between sex and
love, I think their answers would have varied quite a bit
from year to year. We've been through a period of
dramatic changes in sexual mores and sex roles since
that day in the fifties when I first said "I don't believe
it" to the world-wise classmate who tried to explain it to
me.

There's been so much change, in fact, that most

men don't know quite what to think any more. You see the question in every men's magazine: "What do women want?" The question is troublesome because the answer changes so much. When we first began trying to give women what they wanted (and for years before that), they wanted a MAN—in capital letters. They wanted to have their dinners paid for, their chairs held, their doors opened, their cooking complimented, their virginity preserved, and their rings quickly—or so we thought.

Then, suddenly, about the time I was in college, things began to change. In what seemed like only a matter of days, women wanted none of the above. Instead, they wanted free sex, no children, equal pay, our places in law and medical schools, and our jobs afterward. Like many men around me, I thought these new demands were completely reasonable and even welcomed them. Not all men agreed; but conveniently, not all women wanted men who agreed.

So after years of searching for romance and putting women on pedestals, men tried to adjust to years of coping with competition and relating as equals. For many of us, it hasn't been an easy transition. Sex—durable human need that it is—survived pretty well. In some ways, it flourished under the new, looser standards: swinging singles, open marriages, cohabitation. If nothing else, the lack of standards really tested our sexual inventiveness.

But what happened to romance? What happened to candlelit dinners and lovers' lanes and one dozen roses? Unfortunately, most of these were seen by many women as unwelcome reminders of the days when they were considered subordinate ornaments, playthings, amusements. Like millions of men, I caught hell from a woman I liked because I was "romantic"—in the old sense. I learned my lesson, although I was never completely comfortable with it; I tried to stop thinking in terms of romance. I had real trouble, though, when a woman I was involved with told me to treat her "like you would a man." At that point, I was completely lost.

I discovered that the dilemma of the modern man extended into bed. The things I once thought really pleased a woman—taking the initiative, caressing her, pleasing her in every way I knew how—suddenly seemed "sexist"—a strange insult in this context. Nothing was immune to question: positions, techniques, timing, roles, jokes, even fantasies. For a while it seemed as if romance, and with it love, was going to desert even the bed.

During the last ten years or so, I've met dozens of men who were touched by this problem. I've had friends call me in the middle of the night when their partners stalked out of the bedroom because of something they said or did, or something they didn't say or do. I've spent long nights with groups of guys when the only topic of discussion was what women *really* wanted. I've seen the sun rise on these conversations without any satisfactory answers.

The problem, of course, is that these conversations were with the wrong people. That realization struck home when a woman I know pointed out Alexandra Penney's book, *How to Make Love to a Man*. It's based on hundreds of interviews with *men*. The mistake was obvious: we should have been talking to women about how men should make love to them.

HOW TO MAKE LOVE TO A WOMAN

With the help of Steve Naifeh and Greg Smith, I began to talk with every woman I could find who was willing to talk about sex and love. Some of them I knew well, some of them were just friends of friends, most were complete strangers. It didn't matter. Every scrap of information was useful.

What we discovered in hundreds of interviews— some just a few minutes long, some lasting all day and all night, some conducted in person, many others over the telephone—is that women are confused too. Years of changing values, from sorority dances to office romance, have left *them* dizzy too. Many women aren't even sure any more what they're looking for in sex.

Many feel "liberated" and think that the women's movement has been good for women. It has shown them what it means to be an independent person, an equal person, and a "whole" person. But they really aren't sure what role sex is supposed to play in a liberated, "whole" woman's life. How can a woman be "equal"—and still be different in bed? What does it mean to be feminine—or masculine? Does it have to do with attitude, with sex roles, or is anatomy the only difference? What happens to sex when women *and* men are liberated from their traditional sexual roles? These are important questions, and many people—men and women alike—still aren't sure of the answers.

After talking to many, many women, one thing was clear. Women simply aren't interested in sex without love. They want men who are emotionally involved; men who show their concern—before, during, and after sex. They want men who understand that sex is both

4

giving and getting, mutual generosity *and* mutual gratification. Young or old, career woman or housewife, married or single, the women I've talked to want more than sex. They want to make love—and they want to be made love to.

Romance has returned. Or maybe, as one woman suggested, it never really left, but just went underground for a while. All those things men used to do in the fifties and laughed at in the sixties and forgot in the seventies are suddenly reappearing in women's fantasies: candlelight, flowers, music, gifts, dinners, boat rides, dancing, courting, complimenting, confiding, caring. I've heard women talk about all of them as if they're rediscovering a lost and much-missed world.

But there is a difference. The women I've talked to don't wish for a return to the fifties. They are bright, highly independent women. Many of them have careers they consider important, satisfying parts of their lives. Whether their "liberation" has taken place at the office or at home, the lessons of the women's movement have not been lost on these women.

No. Most of them want to be "complete" women, and they want a man to respect that completeness, even in his lovemaking. As one woman said to me, "Sex is something you do with an organ. *Love* is something you do with a person. Love is feeling close emotionally even when you don't feel like having sex. Love is having *better* sex because you *do* feel close emotionally. Love is what I want."

The women's liberation movement taught me and most of the men I know an important lesson. But it wasn't a lesson about equality. Who in the second half of the twentieth century really believes that women are "inferior"? The real lesson of the movement was about *potential*. We learned that women have potentialities that we had never really recognized. They can be executives just as easily as secretaries, managers as easily as mothers, lovers as easily as ladies. Women haven't changed, but our *conception* of women and what women can do has changed dramatically.

The problem is that women are still women, and they still have women's needs. Men have made the mistake of thinking that women are different than they used to be—more like men—when, in fact, they're just *more* than they used to be. Men have mistaken sexual equality for sexual uniformity.

A deluded friend of mine who was having a run of bad luck with women told me, "I like liberated women. You don't have to worry about them. They take care of themselves. It's the best of both worlds: You get the no-pressure business of a buddy and you get the sex too." I told him that with that attitude, I wasn't surprised his luck was bad.

"Equal" doesn't mean "same." And most women I know are quick to point that out. Even a feminist I know says, "A woman can hold down a responsible job, make as much money as her husband or lover, and still be feminine in bed." The lesson is clear: Just because you respect a woman doesn't mean that you can't make love to her.

Yet many liberated women complain that men are now too intimidated to take the aggressive role. At the first sight of a woman in a position of authority, men have abandoned their traditional role of authority in bed. "Even to open a door for a woman," says a male friend, "is inviting disaster. Women see it as a remnant of a banned stereotype. I personally have been yelled at for holding a chair for a woman. I know better now."

Ironically, women are as upset as men about what has happened to sex roles. "The only men who look at me on the streets are foreigners," says another friend. "The American men look right past me—they're afraid I'll be offended. That's not just a guess, either. I've talked to a lot of men who tell me they're afraid of being put down as male chauvinists. I think a lot of liberated women are unhappy sexually. We don't like what we've done to men. I mean, we've made them afraid of their own sexual shadow."

Recognizing the full potential of women doesn't have to mean giving up old sex roles. That's not just wishful thinking from a man who enjoys the old roles, either. During the 1940s, an anthropologist named Frank Beach went to Africa to study primitive cultures in which the occupational roles of men and women were reversed. The women went out in the fields and tilled the soil, provided food, and protected the village. The men stayed home, tended to household chores, and raised the children.

Dr. Beach wanted to know what happened when these people made love. What he found surprised him. Regardless of what they did during the day, at night, for the most part, the women played "feminine" roles, and the men played "masculine" roles. By that, I mean that the men generally played the aggressive role in initiating and carrying through the sex act.

HOW TO MAKE LOVE TO A WOMAN

The time is ripe to reassess the lovemaking act, and the roles that men and women play in it. The time is ripe to reaffirm that, once again, it's right for a man to make love to a woman. If you ask a hundred women what they want from sex in the eighties, ninety-nine will tell you they want a return to romance, a return to wooing and courtship, a return to traditional sex roles and the warmth and intimacy that these can bring.

"All I know about the future," says a C.U.N.Y. student just emerging into full womanhood in the early eighties, "is that I want to love and be loved. I want a man to be a man to me and I want to be a woman to him. And, believe me, I plan to enjoy it."

This book is about a return to romance. This book is about making love.

TWO

No More Macho, No More Wimp

I recently spent an evening with Suzanne, a woman I knew in college. We've seen each other every so often when she comes from her home in Washington to New York on business. Like me, she hasn't married yet.

We were having dinner at a small Indian restaurant when she asked me what I was doing. I told her I was writing a book on how to make love to a woman. She smiled a great big smile and said, "Tell me about it." I did, and she listened with interest, the smile lingering on her lips and occasionally opening up into a big, charming laugh.

"What are you writing about now?" she asked me.

"About women's liberation, and the effect it's had on sex," I said. Most of the guys I know—and women too—who believe in the movement, don't know how to act toward each other. They're always afraid they'll do something sexist."

"I think you're just looking at it from a man's point of view," Suzanne said, without a hint of condescension. "The problem isn't women's liberation so much, it's *men's* liberation. Most of the women I know feel comfortable being women and being equals. It's men who are having trouble adjusting.

"In fact, Betty Friedan just wrote a book called *The Second Stage.*" She pulled a book out of her canvas bag. (Suzanne was always annoyingly resourceful.) "It's not about women's liberation, it's about men's liberation.

"Listen to this. She describes men as 'awkward, isolated, and confused.' That's certainly right for a start. 'With all the attention on the women's movement these past fifteen years,' she goes on, 'it hasn't been noticed that many of the old bases for men's identity have become shaky. If being a man is defined, for example, as being *dominant, superior,* as *not-being-a-woman,* that definition becomes an illusion hard to maintain when most of the important work of society no longer requires brute muscular force . . . . The trouble is, once they disengage themselves from the old patterns of American masculinity and success—John Wayne, Charles Lindbergh, Jack Kennedy—men today are just as lost for lack of role models as women are.'"

Suzanne looked up from the book. Is it sexist, I wondered, to still be fixated on large blue eyes? "This is especially interesting," she went on. "Friedan says that, in their fear and confusion, men have retreated from masculinity altogether. 'Deluged with sexual information from the mass media, they [women] *notice,* and even say so, when their men are not good lovers. Men, who used to be the measure of all things, may indeed shrivel up or flee from the experience of being measured themselves.' Sounds pretty pessimistic, huh?"

What else could I do but nod?

"But you'd be surprised how optimistic her predictions are. She says the women's movement was really a people's movement, and the result is going to be a society in which all people—men and women alike— feel free to express a whole range of emotions, from strength and self-confidence to gentleness and vulnerability. It'll be wide open and everybody will benefit.

"She says, 'Now men as well as women are asking for real intimacy, sharing, *feelings* . . . . It seems strange to suggest that there is a new American frontier, a new adventure for men, in this new struggle for *wholeness*, for openness to feeling, for living and sharing life on equal terms with women . . . the human liberation that began with the women's movement.'

"Aren't you glad," she said, smoothing back her hair, "we're alive today?

"Now," she said with a laugh, "let's eat. The tambouri is getting cold."

When we were finished, she said with authority, "I'll pay the bill. Remember, I invited you." But when we got up, she looked at me with a shy smile, and said: "Would you help me with my coat?"

My conversation with Suzanne and other women since have confirmed the view that the return of sex roles in the eighties won't be a return to stereotypes or stereotyped sex. The 1960s and 1970s were a period of consciousness-raising. We now know that women can show strength and still be feminine, and that men can be gentle and still be masculine. We know that women have always enjoyed taking an active role in bed from time to time. We also know that men enjoy giving up the lead from time to time. Making love is a *shared* responsibility.

The popularity of *How to Make Love to a Man* underlined this, as did the 1975 *Redbook* poll, the largest poll ever on women's sexuality. A questionnaire consisting of sixty items was published and almost 100,000 replies were received. (The famous 1953 Kinsey study, *Sexual Behavior in the Human Female*, was based on fewer than 8,000 replies.)

The *Redbook* poll revealed that six out of ten wives say they initiate sex at least half the time; nine out of ten say they take an active part during lovemaking at least half the time (and four of the nine say they are always active). An even more startling revelation: less than 1 percent of the women are sexually completely passive. Women want to share the responsibility of lovemaking.

Unfortunately, despite all the polls and all the studies, the two sexual stereotypes that women would be happiest to see die are still held by some men—even though most are afraid to admit it. The first is that a woman wants a man to set her on a pedestal (the "Pedestal Syndrome"). The second is that a woman wants to be taken or possessed by force (the "Possession Syndrome").

Many men think both of these stereotypes are the products of women's fantasies. That idea is a male fantasy of its own. But even if they were what women wanted, they'd still have nothing to do with making love to a woman. A woman is not an object to be venerated, nor is she a possession to be taken by brute force. She's a human being. She has human sensibilities, including a sense of privacy that is violated by any uninvited intrusions; and human drives, including a normal sexual appetite that needs to be satisfied.

The Pedestal Syndrome

The Pedestal Syndrome probably originated in the chivalrous romances of the Middle Ages. Women remained shut up in tall fortresses, mostly doing needlework, while their knights—literally in shining armor—competed for their favor. The Guineveres of the world were supposed to remain untouched until the proper moment. At the first hint that their purity had been compromised by an errant Lancelot, the Arthurs of the period flew into fits of panic and fury.

The amazing thing is not that the Pedestal Syndrome developed in a time of distinct sexual roles, but that it has survived the fading of those roles.

"I always wondered whether women were really interested in sex," says a professional football player in Dallas. "My first wife was the sweetest, most feminine woman I ever met. I always thought she just put up with sex until I overheard her talking to her old college roommates. You should have heard them. I mean, one of them was saying, 'I really like to have a man come in my mouth.' The others were all saying, 'Ooh, I *hate* that!' Sex-talk, graphic stuff, worse than any locker room I've been in."

Another woman told me about a friend of hers who performed oral sex on her husband for the first time a few weeks after they were married. He pulled away, irate, saying, "Where did you learn that?"

In a recent poll of American high-school students, between 60 and 70 percent of the male students said they would prefer to marry a virgin. That should tell you something. Most men want someone with little or no sexual experience. Someone who'll let *them* be the teacher. Why do they want to be teachers? Because teachers make the rules and set the limits.

The cat is finally out of the bag: women *do* want sex. They not only know about it, they enjoy it. It's not beneath them, it doesn't "dirty" them, defile them, or damage them. Woman are not delicate creatures who require special care and handling like rare tropical flowers. And, equally important, they don't need a teacher to teach them the steps or make the rules.

One problem with putting a woman on a pedestal is that the pedestal becomes shaky when she finally decides to let go and make love. I knew a guy named George who fell in love regularly and pursued women on a career basis. George treated women like goddesses. He would come to my apartment and spend hours telling me about the perfection of his latest Aphrodite. He would send flowers to her almost daily (George was rich), take her to expensive restaurants, plays, discos, etc. Within two weeks, he was usually talking about marriage.

But within three or four weeks, the affair was always over. Why? Because by the third or fourth week, George had usually been able to coax his goddess into bed. And once George had slept with a woman, he lost all interest in her. What interested him was winning a woman, not the woman herself, and winning her brought his interest to an end. By the next day, he would start wondering why he had ever found her attractive. Out of the corner of his eye—even before he had broken off the old affair—the search for a new Aphrodite would begin.

Women are not the only victims of the Pedestal Syndrome. The act of love itself is cheapened for the man by the idea that women are pure and sex will somehow "spoil" them. When a man loses respect for the woman he sleeps with, sex is hardly an intimate and positive experience for him or for the woman.

There's a time in the life of every woman when she wants to be truly courted—placed on a pedestal, you might say. But the same can be said for most men. "Who doesn't want somebody, sometime, somewhere, to think that they're the best thing that ever happened to the world," says one woman. "I don't mind a man putting me on a pedestal—so long as he doesn't leave me there."

The Possession Syndrome

Like the Pedestal Syndrome, the Possession Syndrome probably got its start during the Middle Ages. At that time, the reason for rape was not lust but greed. A man raped another man's woman for the same reason that he stole his money: to establish ownership. Rape was theft of another man's property.

"This property notion still affects women," says a female history professor at a small eastern liberal arts college. "When a woman wants to remain a virgin, she's accepting both the religious notion that premarital sex is immoral, and the cultural notion that she's the property of her future husband. In a way, being possessed a little against her will is a shortcut out of that dilemma. Then she gets the sex but she hasn't done anything herself to bring it about. She avoids the taboos."

Many women will reluctantly admit that the Possession Syndrome has some basis in female fantasies. "But," says a female doctor in Boston, "men have blown it *way* out of proportion. They've made it into a fulfillment of their own fantasies of violence and domination."

For most women, the so-called desire to be raped takes two forms—neither of which has anything to do with the crime called rape. To some women, it's a license to be passive, an expression of the occasional desire to be dominated, manipulated, and controlled.

For some women, possession fantasies are just playacting. "Sometimes my husband and I decide that he's going to 'take' me. He throws me on the bed, pulls my clothes off, you know, forces me to do things. Sometimes I even pretend to make a fuss, put up a fight, resist him, that sort of thing. But for God's sake, that certainly doesn't mean I want to be raped. God forbid I should ever be raped. There's nothing Freudian about it. There's nothing neurotic about it. It's just out-in-the-open fantasy and playacting. Playacting's just another way for us to enjoy sex." If a woman you're with suggests playacting a rape fantasy, just remember that there's an important line between fantasy and reality.

Of course, men feel this desire occasionally too—the desire to be taken care of in an aggressive physical way. "It seems silly to call it rape," says a male friend of mine, "but I do like to be 'manhandled' by a woman sometimes. The best way to do it is to pretend you're really tired, too tired to move. You both know it's kind of a joke, but it gives me a chance to be completely submissive."

"In most relationships today," says one young woman, "the one who takes the initiative is the one with the bigger libido. I know women with monster sex drives who are afraid to take the initiative because they're afraid the guy will be offended. I can see that. A lot of guys lose it when you're in the mood and they're not. It frightens them. But once you're *in* bed, and you're both in the mood, I think guys get off on a little aggressiveness."

"There are no pat answers," sums up a Los Angeles woman. "Some women want to swing from the rafters, some want to lie there like mannequins. I want both— one one night, the other the next night. It all depends— on the woman, on the man, on the mood."

Only one thing doesn't depend. Nothing is more of an obstacle to good lovemaking than stereotypes. When a man makes love according to stereotypes, he's denying that a woman has any needs of her own. He's saying to her: "You're not a person, you're a gender, a type. I care more about having sex with a woman than about making love to you." In the eighties, making love by stereotypes is not making love at all.

One woman said it all in one pointed remark. "I think the title's wrong," she said when I told her about the book. "It should be *How to Make Love* with *a Woman*."

THREE

What Women Find Sexy in a Man

If you asked men at random what women find sexy in men, you would get answers like: "They're all looking for Paul Newman," or "a good build," or "impressive equipment—a man who has a lot and knows how to use all of it." I know because I asked, and those are some of the answers I got. They're also *typical* of the answers.

Another widespread male myth is that a man who can "perform" like a "stud stallion" is a real turn-on for women. Like most myths, this one misses the mark. Most women don't find the ability to perform like a "stud" attractive. Performance isn't even on the list.

What women *really* find sexy in a man is, of course, a different story entirely. When I asked random women the same question, the answer was almost always the same. The single most attractive thing about a man is self-assurance. Actually, this shouldn't come as a complete surprise. Alexandra Penney states in her book that men put self-confidence at the top of the list of desirable attributes in women.

Although some women say good looks is a turn-on, they're decidedly in the minority. A more typical response was, "I don't like really good-looking men. They're so into themselves, they don't have anything left over for someone else." Another said, "You don't need Robert Redford. You need someone who has a 'gestalt' quality." And another, "I don't give a damn what they look like. I care about energy. Someone without energy is a total turn-off for me."

"A nice healthy ego is easily the most important thing," says a middle-aged businesswoman. "Of course, any woman is attracted to a man who's handsome. But every woman knows there's no relationship between how a man looks and how he loves. At one time or another, we've all gone gaga over a real looker only to find out he's gay, or gone home with someone who's five-foot-six—and looks like he spent his life in the public library—only to discover that he's thunder in bed."

Why do women want one thing and men think they want something else? Why isn't communication any better? The experts who study communication between men and women (or lack of it) think that it works like a self-fulfilling prophecy.

Men who *think* that women are looking for good features—a good physique, or oversized penises—but who don't have them, will lack self-esteem. The women are turned off, not by the physical attributes (or lack of them), but by the lack of self-confidence. The men, of course, detect the turn-off and just figure it's because they don't have the necessary physical attributes. "It's a real circle," says a Los Angeles therapist. "And nobody wins."

The most important part of a man's ability to make love is his attitude toward himself. If a man basically likes himself, if he feels comfortable with his body, comfortable with other people, and relaxed around women, he is "sexy" in the eyes of ninety-nine out of a hundred women. And that's true regardless of his features, his pectorals, or his pecker.

One woman put it pointedly: "What's sexy? That's easy. If he thinks he's sexy, he's sexy."

What man hasn't heard the old saying that the ultimate aphrodisiac for women is power. Don't we all have fantasies of being rich and powerful, or rich and famous, and getting anything we want from any woman we want? Gossip columnists in Washington papers are filled with stories of the wayward ways of senators and congressmen who slip from one extramarital affair to the next with women half their ages and twice their I.Q.'s.

An attractive female assistant to a midwestern congressman talking with me about the sexual goings-on on Capitol Hill admitted in confidence that she, like a lot of women in her position, knew her boss "intimately."

"What is it about him that turns you on?" I asked. "He's certainly no matinee idol."

She reflected for a moment. "He's so sure of himself," she finally said. "The men I used to date were always worried about their images. I spent the whole day—and every night—massaging their egos. The sex was like therapy. *These* men are different. Their egos are in great shape. They don't worry about themselves as much. They worry about me and my ego. That's a nice thing."

A middle-aged woman in Dallas said she'd had it with insecure men: "I feel like I'm constantly running around with a basket trying to catch the balls they throw in the air. You have to be so protective of their manhood. You have to make them feel stronger and bigger and smarter than you are. I spent all my time trying to be less than the men I was involved with. That's why I like the rare man who's secure in his manhood. And that *doesn't* mean macho men. Macho men—men who swagger around and *tell* you how masculine they are—aren't secure in their masculinity at all."

One thing women are unanimous about is their distaste for *over*confidence. "The Cult of the Lady-Killer," as one woman calls it, is probably the most misguided male myth of all. It's the product of a complete breakdown in communication between men and women. It's a distillation of everything men *think* women want—but, in fact, most women loathe.

"There's nothing more obnoxious than a so-called Don Juan," says a woman who works at Tiffany's in New York. "If he acts like a seducer, you end up wondering to yourself, 'How many other people has he pulled these lines on?' I'm not interested in becoming the latest link in a long chain. I don't want someone who wants to make love for its own sake—to show what a great lover he is. I want someone who wants to make love to *me*."

What are the turn-ons? Some are physical characteristics; some are psychological. Either way, they're within reach of most men. In other words, they're things you can do something about.

A Sexy Body

Eyes

If you asked a group of men what part of a woman's body was the biggest turn-on, you might get a hundred different answers, but the two big winners would be breasts and legs. Women also seem to break down into two groups: eye-lookers and ass-lookers. In a recent *Esquire* poll, eyes ranked as the sexiest part of a man's body; asses took second place. (In most polls, hands ranked third.)

"Oh, that's easy," said a tall brunette without blinking when I asked her the same question. "The first thing I look at is his eyes. One look in a man's eyes and I know right away if I'm interested."

What precisely is it about the eyes, I asked, that turned her on. "What kind of eyes do you like?"

"Oh, brown, I guess, or blue. What's really important is what they *say* to me."

Women who are eye-lookers uniformly believe that the eyes speak a language of their own. They believe they can read a man's whole character in his eyes. They can tell if he's gentle or strong, lustful or loving, callous or caring.

"It's all in the eye contact," explains a woman doctor in Pittsburgh. "If his eyes dart around and avoid you nervously, that's a sure sign he's not very self-confident. A man who can't sustain eye contact with a woman is a washout—with me, at least."

An actor and writer I know in New York has a way of focusing on the woman he's with, even if they're in a crowded room. During a conversation, he rests his elbow on the table and puts his hand to his brow as if shielding his eyes from the sun. What he's really doing is focusing his attention on her—shielding out any distractions. He's creating a circle of exclusivity. He's saying to the woman: "In this room, right now, you're the only thing that matters to me."

Remember that your eyes are the part of your body that can convey that message most convincingly—whether you're in a crowd or alone in bed.

Physique

The New York *Village Voice* recently polled a large sample of women asking the same question: What part of a man's body turns women on most? Contrary to the *Esquire* poll, the landslide winner was the ass. Coming in a distant second was a "flat stomach." If you think about it, you'll see what good news that is. Asses and stomachs, unlike bone structure and penis size, are things you can do something about. An ass can be tightened and a stomach flattened with some regular exercise and, if you're serious, a routine at a local gym.

Don't get me wrong. If your sex life is the problem, pumping iron isn't the answer. Many women are turned off by too much muscle.

But if you're uncertain about your physical appearance, two trips a week to a gym will give your self-confidence a boost. In fact, they'll do more for you than assurances from a woman that she likes your looks. "Trips to the gym," says a middle-aged lawyer in Chicago who's a "born-again" athlete, "do more for me than a weekly trip to the psychiatrist—and they're cheaper."

The confidence comes from getting back in touch with your body. "I never really liked sports," said the same man, showing off his washboard stomach. "I was like a stranger in my own body, but I didn't care. But, boy, what a difference it makes with sex. Before I started to work out, I used to make love with my cock. It was as if my cock was the only part of me that was in bed.

Now I'm back in touch with my body and when I have an orgasm, my whole body, every part of me, feels it."

Grooming

I'm not sure whether women are turned *on* by a well-groomed man, or just turned *off* by sloppy grooming. Either way, it amounts to the same thing. That doesn't mean you should look flawless. Many, many women are turned off by men who worry about their looks, primp constantly, and can't pass a mirror without a sidelong glance. It's definitely possible to be *too* well-groomed. Women consider that kind of preoccupation with appearance much too self-conscious, perhaps even unmanly.

So, take time in front of the mirror, just not too much. "I don't want a slob, of course," says a secretary from Seattle. "But when a guy is really conscious of his looks, I can't help thinking that he's too conscious of *my* appearance. You know, examining every detail of me to see if I measure up to him. It makes me nervous."

Some odors are pleasing to some women, but offensive to others. Tobacco and alcohol, for example. It's up to you to figure out how she reacts and deal with it accordingly. If you're an inveterate smoker, you may have to choose between cigarettes and her. It's almost impossible to disguise the smell of cigarettes on the breath of a regular smoker.

Colognes are in the category of smells that some women like and some don't. But most women tend to think that a slight, natural masculine scent is more sexy. "I'm sort of embarrassed to say it," one woman revealed, "but a slight body odor actually turns me on. It's definitely an aphrodisiac. Of course, too much is a different story."

Another woman, a television actress working in New York, told me that she once "fell in love with a man because of the way he smelled. I was constantly leaning on his shoulder and trying to smell him. We used to fight like crazy. But when he got close to me, I'd swoon. Some people just smell sexy."

Tone of Voice

Women are much more sexually attuned to men's voices than men are to women's voices. Many women find a sexy voice one of a man's most powerful turn-ons. One attractive woman I know cares more about a man's voice than anything else. She's indifferent to good looks, muscles, power, money, and all the more traditional aphrodisiacs. But, as she says, "Put me in the arms of a man with a deep, husky baritone in a dark room and I'm putty."

A Sexy Mind

Real self-confidence starts in your mind and radiates out into your body. On careful reflection, the vast majority of the women I spoke with said the sexiest man is a man with a "sexy mind." When I asked them what that meant, several phrases kept cropping up: widespread interests, wide-ranging intellect, good sense of humor, charming conversational manner, and the ability to make a woman feel that she's the only thing that matters.

Intelligence and Charm

A leading woman's magazine recently published an article about the men that women "dream about"—the men they find sexy. Some of the lucky chosen were predictable: "jocks" like Bruce Jenner and Joe Namath, "tough guys" like Charles Bronson and Larry Hagman, "heart-throbs" like Richard Gere and Marcello Mastroianni.

But men with physical attributes didn't dominate the list. It also included "Ivy Leaguers" like actor Michael Moriarty and cartoonist Gary Trudeau, "intellectuals" like columnist William Buckley and novelist John Updike, even "irresistible lunatics" like Woody Allen. Obviously, if Woody Allen is being listed as one of the sexiest men in America, American women are not attracted to good looks alone.

Woody Allen has another characteristic women find sexy: a sense of humor. Says a student at a large midwestern state university: "The only guy I want to spend a long time with is one who can make me laugh."

And from another: "Artists are sexy. They're uninhibited and experimental. They bring their creativity to sex. You never know what they're going to do next. I've had a lot of sex in my life, but I had a strict religious upbringing, and you never lose that sense of prudishness. It takes an uninhibited man to break down my inhibitions."

Paying Attention

"I like Italian men the best," offered a striking blond

real-estate agent in San Francisco. "Once Italians leave the office, they stop thinking about their work. When you make love to some men, you know you're making love to someone who wants to make a business deal the next morning. You only get half of them. Half of them are already thinking about the deal.

"Italian men—their entire need is focused on the woman. They may not speak to you the next day, but during the lovemaking you're the only thing on their minds. They touch a lot. Italian men seem consumed by a woman's body. They take their time with her, they spend hours fondling her. The time before sex is a special, almost spiritual event for them. They're in tune with their animal natures—but they aren't tough. In fact, Italian men are exceptionally gentle."

What can you do to free your mind of all distractions—to concentrate your attention on the woman you're with? How can you clear your mind of the problems of the day so you can experience the pleasures of the moment?

A thirty-five-year-old actor who often appears in Broadway shows once let me in on a remarkable method of preparing for an evening of lovemaking. "An hour or so before I go out with a woman," he said, "I sit down calmly for a few minutes and run the evening across the screen of my imagination. It's sort of like a preview of what's to come."

The advantage of thinking about what's going on in her mind is that it will help you concentrate all of your attention on her when you see her—not just on her body, but on *her*, her life, her desires, her excitements, her needs. As one woman put it, "The man who turns me on is the man who's interested in me." That *concentrated* attention is one of the things women find sexiest in a man.

A Man Who Likes Women

If anything startled me in my discussions with the women I interviewed, it was the frequent comment that most men basically—if subconsciously—don't like women. They may want women for sex, but not for friends. And even if they're not aware of it, the women usually are.

"I think many American men don't like women," said one young writer in Boston. "Now, I don't feel they have it out for women or anything. I just think American men feel uncomfortable with intimacy. When they're with their close male friends, they concentrate on joint activities. They go out and play some basketball, or go fishing, or go out for some beers, or watch the baseball game, or whatever. They *don't* talk about their troubles, especially their emotional and sexual troubles. Women talk about those issues all the time, and they expect the same kinds of intimacy from the men in their lives. Since women are demanding levels of warmth and intimacy that the men in their lives simply aren't capable of producing, the men begin to resent them—however unconsciously."

Said another: "They think we aren't trustworthy. That we're trying to get something from them. I think a lot of them didn't like their mothers, and they project that dislike on the women they know. Men who really like women are joked about. I like men who can joke the way women can. And that doesn't mean someone who's effeminate.

"The problem is just that most men don't grow up

with a vocabulary for intimacy—or for personal things. When they talk with close male friends, they talk about sports and different things. Women learn the words. Men are frustrated because of the lack of an adequate vocabulary. That's why I'm so surprised—and so delighted—when I actually meet a man who obviously enjoys being with women and talking about the kinds of things women talk about."

One woman probably put it best when she said, "A sexy man is a man who obviously *likes* women. Someone who enjoys their company. Not all men do, you know, and you can tell it immediately." Another woman meant the same thing when she said, "Men should learn to be friends with women. They can make such *good* friends. The best sex is sex between two friends."

Passion

Another quality women look for in men is passion, passion for life, of course, and for love. A college professor in Maryland told me she always looked for a man with "a zest for life." "If a man has a lot of interests and enthusiasms," she said, "he'll be enthusiastic in his relationship with me." Why is a zest for life so important? "I guess it's because a man who is enthusiastic about life generally is sure of himself. He has a healthy ego—and that's always good for me too."

And from still another woman: "Sexy men are men who feel passionate about everything that they do. They're capable of extremes of feeling. Their feeling toward life spills over into sex. If a man is bored with his career, he won't be able to summon up the passion to be a great lover. The best come-on is a man's passion. No woman is immune to it."

FOUR

Fears of Flying

Most men are painfully familiar with sexual fears. I've never met a man who didn't, at one time or another, have some sexual problem—real or imagined—to worry about. This guy's ejaculations are too quick, that guy's erections are "here one minute, gone the next," and there are all of those men out there who have been issued undersized equipment.

In fact, most men are so busy worrying about their own fears that they often don't bother to stop and realize that women have sexual fears, too. The result is misunderstanding and resentment. "I'm tired of playing sexual wet nurse to men," says one woman. "It seems like I spend the whole night saying, 'No, no, that's okay. No, it was good. No, size doesn't matter.' You know, all that bullshit. I'm not alone, either. I know a lot of other women who don't like playing Florence Nightingale of the Bedroom."

If neither partner is willing to play the nurse role and help the other deal with his or her sexual fears, then what you really have is two ships passing each other in a fog—a fog of misunderstanding and ignorance. The only way out of that fog is to try to see sex and love from the other's perspective. Many men have never stopped to ask themselves what it is about sex that a woman enjoys most—or fears most. Yet you can't begin to make real love to a woman without knowing what makes her happy—and what makes her afraid.

In one way at least, a woman's sexual anxieties are like a man's. They're based on a fear of rejection. Almost every man I know has felt rejected by a woman. Sometimes that rejection is real, but more often it's just the result of ignorance. If a woman isn't aware of a man's sexual fears, she can send him a message of rejection without ever meaning to.

Men do the same thing to women, maybe even more often because they aren't used to the idea that women *have* sexual fears. And, again, the message is often unintended. By learning more about a woman's sexual fears, a man can know when he should take the time to reassure her and to dispel her fear of rejection.

"I'm not attractive enough."

A classmate of mine at law school constantly talked about women's looks. He'd go through the first-year class giving each girl a rating from one to ten. As we walked down the hall, he would recite a steady stream of numbers: "Eight. Six. Four—she's a real loser. Wow—a definite nine and a half."

No wonder so many women spend so much time worrying about how attractive they are: "Am I pretty enough? Do I need to lose a few pounds? Will he see my stretch marks? Isn't my cellulite ugly? Am I too old? Should I have a nose job? I don't look anything like the girls in *Playboy!*" Even the prettiest women tend to be blinded to their own beauty by a preoccupation with the inevitable flaw. The number-one female fear, especially among younger women, is "I'm not attractive enough."

What they don't understand is that much of the talk about women's looks is just that—talk. When it comes to love, most of the men I know really aren't as hung up about physical appearance as they say they are. While young men—especially when they're still in school and subject to peer pressure—may seem preoccupied with a woman's face or body, that hangup fades as the looking gets more serious. As they mature, they tend to lose their interest in the "mirror" virtues and start looking for other attributes.

What mature men really find attractive is not perfect features or a twenty-two-inch waist, it's a woman who feels at home with herself. In fact, eight out of ten men in another *Redbook* survey said they were more excited by "a woman who loves me" than by large breasts or any of the other macho turn-ons. The problem is that most women don't know that. If men would only let women in on this little secret, a lot of women would feel a lot easier about having sex.

So let her know that she's appealing to you. "If a man makes a woman feel beautiful or sexy," says a woman I know, "it's the damnedest thing, but she *becomes* much more beautiful. She loses her self-consciousness and the sex gets real good."

By the way, I recently met up with my law-school friend. He had married one of our classmates, he announced happily. He asked me if I remembered her and I did. I also remembered that he had rated her a "definite five and a half."

"My breasts are too small (or too large)."

"Girls growing up don't have penis envy," a friend in Boston told me. "They have breast envy. They spend at least as much time sizing each other up in the locker room as men do. By the time they've grown up and begun having sex, they approach each new sexual partner anxious that they won't 'measure up.'"

If a woman's breasts are "too" large or "too" small—meaning that she *thinks* they're too large or too small—you need to let her know that you appreciate them as they are.

If you're one of the many men who *prefer* small breasts, let your partner know that; it will put her at ease. Many men prefer women who are active athletically, and they often have smaller breasts.

In fact, there's no such thing as a breast that's "too" small. Forget those Hollywood visions of forty-two-inch busts. Breasts that big are rare, frequently faked or silicone-induced, awkward in lovemaking, and often, almost numb to the touch. Remember, the goal is to give your partner pleasure, not measure her against this month's pinup.

If you think a woman is very sensitive about the size of her breasts, don't bring up the subject—even to reassure her. (If a woman said to you, "It's okay, I like small penises," would it make you feel better?) Where anxieties are involved, actions always speak louder than words.

"He's using me."

No matter how "liberated" a woman is, the fear of exploitation remains strong. Women who have freed themselves from the feeling that men will lose respect for them if they have sex are still concerned that the act of lovemaking might be somehow "trivialized." As one woman said, "Even if it's just for one night, it should *matter*." The fear that it (sex, lovemaking) won't matter is probably rooted in the older fear of being treated like an object. Many women who have no moral objection to frequent sex say they feel somehow "cheapened" by it if it's just sex for sex's sake.

When it comes to sex, many women are still living in two worlds. There's the world they grew up in and the world of today. The first predates the sexual revolution; the second is its product. The conflict between these two worlds, and their wildly different attitudes toward sex, produces one of the most profound of women's sexual anxieties.

"People my age grew up believing you had to date someone four or five months before it was okay to 'do it,'" says a forty-five-year-old divorcee in Tulsa, Oklahoma. "Sure, I believe in the sexual revolution. My mind believes it. My body believes it. My *heart* just doesn't believe. It keeps holding out. As a girl, they told me, if I gave in, he'd never respect me. I guess I still feel that way, all these years later."

Unfortunately, men haven't made the situation any easier. Despite all the talk of sexual revolution, many men are still in prerevolutionary days when it comes to *women* having sex. Many men still *don't* respect women who have sex outside wedlock, or at the very least, outside a long-term relationship. This is easy to see in the Don Juan who stops seeing a woman as soon as he's finally gotten her into bed. But many men who might deny it put inordinate emphasis on the conquest and make women as a group wary.

Although some men express similar reservations about indiscriminate sex, it is more of an anxiety for women. Somehow, more seems to be at stake for them, particularly in relationships that aren't exclusive. Typically, a woman doesn't expect a man to make mad, passionate love to her every time. She doesn't have to be his obsession. But she *does* want—*expect*—him to make love to her because he really wants to, because he really *likes* her.

"He'll want me to do something I don't want to do."

Many women, especially inexperienced women, approach the bed with serious anxiety. They're afraid that a man may ask them to do something that they don't know how to do or don't want to do. The main culprit is oral sex.

"Whenever I go to bed with a man for the first few times," a woman in Baltimore told me, "I'm anxious that he'll expect me to do oral sex. I *hate* oral sex. I *hate* it if a man pulls my head down and wants me to do it." Another woman said, "I'm not keen on sucking. I don't mind the sucking but I don't want anyone to come inside my mouth. I also don't like anal sex. I don't think the body was made for that—that's why it hurts. I think it's an angry, aggressive act. It has an edge of violence to it."

The combination of sexual revolution and women's liberation have opened up new vistas of sexual potential for women, and also new responsibilities. Equality has its costs, and fellatio is one of them. Many women find the new freedom more than a little frightening. The best way for a man to deal with a woman's sexual fear is to put himself in her place, to try to feel the way she feels, fear the way she fears.

Think of it this way: In the beginning, she may feel just as uncomfortable about giving you oral sex as you feel about giving her oral sex. You wouldn't want to feel pressured into performing cunnilingus, so you should take care not to pressure her into performing fellatio.

It's up to you to persuade her—through actions, not words—that making love is not passing a test. That she's not going to have to express her feelings for you by doing anything she doesn't want to do. Chances are, if the atmosphere is calm and caring—if you don't pressure her—what she does or doesn't want to do may *change*. When she sees how much you enjoy giving her the pleasure of cunnilingus, for example, eventually she may want to give you the reciprocal pleasure of fellatio.

"I may get pregnant."

In this era of sex education, the Pill, and every kind of contraceptive device, it's hard for men to believe that women are still afraid of unwanted pregnancy. Obviously, this is another place where communication has failed, because woman after woman after woman mentioned the fear of accidental conception.

Some even expressed anger at the seeming lack of

concern among most men: "Most men aren't in the least concerned with what kind of birth control I use. I guess they assume that, if I don't mention it, I'm on the Pill. The few times a man asks me I'm so gratified they *care*— that they care about me as a person. Sometimes, they even say it in an accusatory way—'You're on the Pill, aren't you'—as if I'm trying to *trap* them with a pregnancy."

"I wish we'd known about contraceptives when I first started having sex," said one woman about her loss of virginity twenty years ago. "I spent the next twenty-eight days worried. A few decades ago, most of your life you spent worried."

But the worry really isn't over. "It haunts me," said an attractive brunette in her thirties who is very involved in a banking career. "No matter what precaution you take, you know you're just never *sure*. I stopped taking the Pill because of all the side-effects questions. And nothing else is completely reliable. I keep thinking, 'Oh, God, a baby. What would I do with a baby?'"

The problem of contraception is particularly acute the first time you make love to a woman. You may not be sure if she's on the Pill, and if not, if she's protected. Ways to deal with the problem of contraception the first time you make love to a woman are discussed in detail in chapter 11.

There is no ideal form of contraception. The Pill is the most effective method, but also probably the most dangerous and many women have stopped using it. It can lead to cysts, clotting, and other serious medical problems for the woman. Although no form of

contraceptive is 100 percent effective (even the Pill is
only 99 percent sure) some are less effective than others.
IUDs are bad for several reasons. They have been
known to scar the cervix; they can also be dislodged.
The best contraceptive is probably the diaphragm,
always to be used with some form of spermicidal jelly
inserted no more than two hours before intercourse, and
always to be left in place at least six hours after
intercourse.

If you are in a continuing relationship, and she's not
on the Pill and hasn't worked out some other means of
contraception, recommend that she obtain a diaphragm,
which should not cause any medical problems and
should provide a high degree of protection from
pregnancy. The fear of unwanted pregnancy is one
female fear that you should resolve from the moment a
sexual relationship begins.

"I'll hurt him—or else I'll get hurt."

No one, man or woman, wants to get involved with
someone who is emotionally fragile. That kind of
fragility is the opposite of self-confidence. But no matter
how self-confident a woman is, the fear of rejection
remains.

The other side of getting hurt is hurting. Before, it
was a man's sexual fear that the woman he had sex with
would get too serious too soon. Too much real affection
during sex would send him scurrying for cover. But
equality has changed things, and now women are
beginning to share the same fear.

Maxine Schnall, author of *Limits: A Search for New
Values*, argues that a major problem since the seventies

is what she calls "commitmentphobia." She defines this as "an incapacity to enter into or sustain an exclusive, permanent relationship with a member of the opposite sex. The commitmentphobe has, in essence, become sexually available at the cost of emotional accessibility, making tenderness the new taboo."

While the problem is most commonly male, Schnall finds, women too, are increasingly wary of long-term emotional commitments. Afraid to exhibit vulnerable, "feminine" characteristics, the female commitmentphobe is attracted to inaccessible men—men who will not become dependent on them. Like their male counterparts, they find it difficult to believe that "it is possible to be both autonomous and deeply committed to one another."

A twenty-two-year-old magazine editor in New York says, "Men are much more hung up on sex than we are. If you end the affair, you're afraid you'll give them a hangup for life. So you end up hanging onto awkward relationships when you really don't want to— or else you just avoid them altogether."

The solution seems to be the same whether a woman's fear is getting hurt or hurting. You should be cautious in declaring commitments, or making hints of long-term involvements. Avoiding "I love you" early in a relationship is probably a good idea for two reasons: You'll allay her fears of getting hurt *and* her feelings of hurting you. "People are always so trigger-happy with 'I love you,'" says a friend. "I always remember what John Wayne said in a movie about using a gun: 'Don't shoot unless you mean to kill.'"

If you must see more than one woman at a time,

observe simple etiquette. Let each woman know about the other, but don't talk about the woman you're not with. And remember: the best sex takes place when love is at its best, and the only way to really love a woman is to love her alone.

FIVE

Courtship and Romance

Before the 1960s, American movies were filled with dashing men wooing beautiful women; romance was the crucial prelude to making love. Especially during the depths of the Depression, the silver screen showed the leading men of the time taking their leading ladies to black-tie dinners at elegant restaurants, filling their rooms wall to wall with elaborate flower arrangements, and speaking eloquent words of love on the marble terraces of fabulous mansions, always under a clear sky and in the light of a full moon.

Things have changed, all right. In a recent blockbuster film, John Travolta doesn't even bother to ask the woman's name until *after* they've had sex. No wonder most women believe romance is due for a revival.

One thing hasn't changed, of course: romance is still expensive. Taking the woman you love to one of the truly great restaurants (forget the black tie) can cost a week's wages. The money required to fill her room with flowers could pay your own rent for a month or two.

All the women I spoke with said they expect to be taken out by the men who are wooing them; they said they expect a present from time to time; they long for these signs of caring and affection. Yet most of these signs are very expensive. The practical question for most men is, how can you be romantic without being rich?

Women's liberation or no women's liberation, almost all women expect to be courted. As one career woman in New York put it, "Underneath all those 'dress-for-success' business suits you'll probably find lacy underwear. Don't be misled by a hard-edge business exterior. I still appreciate roses and silly Valentine cards."

But what women expect from courtship varies from one region of the country to another and from one age group to another. Some women expect to share more of the expense of romance than others. At the risk of generalization, women in the southern and southwestern states expect more of their boyfriends and lovers than women elsewhere. In other states, age becomes the primary factor. "If a man is over forty," says a twenty-nine-year-old businesswoman in Chicago, "he generally expects to pay when you go out; if he's under thirty, he generally expects you to share the costs; if he's between thirty and forty, the situation is more flexible."

To find out how to handle those potentially awkward "flexible situations," I asked psychologist Dr. Marilyn Machlowitz about them. "A woman today may be earning almost as much as you—or, perish the thought, even more," said Dr. Machlowitz. "How then do you handle the delicate issue of who picks up the check? Waiters, having been trained and sensitized to this issue, no longer automatically hand it to the man. Instead, they place it in a DMZ in the middle of the table.

"Unless you've made it clear that you're paying when you made the dinner arrangements, what you might do is take the lead. Say, 'How do you want to handle this?' or 'I'm treating you this time, you can take me next time.'

"This succeeds in establishing a couple of things. First, that you value and respect the woman's opinion. Women—and men, too, for that matter—don't like having orders and demands handed to them. Second, it establishes you as gracious and fair. You're not whipping out your pocket calculator and saying, 'You owe me thirteen fifty-two.'"

In the "old days," before romance went out of fashion, men and women often handled the problem of sharing expenses this way: The man would invite the woman out to dinner; the woman would then reciprocate by inviting the man to a home-cooked dinner. There were only a few variations on this theme. She might stick a pizza in the oven, for example, and he would bring the six-pack of beer.

Today, the possibilities for sharing expenses are much more varied. For one thing, she can invite *you* out to dinner, then you can cook dinner for *her* at your place. Most women are moved more by the time that you spend preparing a meal yourself than by the money that you spend paying the restaurant to do it for you.

Or, if she earns as much as you do, you can simply trade off paying the bill; you pay one bill, she pays the next. There is one caveat to the trade-off system, however. If you have invited a woman to an expensive restaurant, you should always plan to pick up the entire tab. It simply isn't fair to invite her to a meal more expensive than she might choose by herself and then expect her to pay half the bill.

However you decide to handle the bill, remember that a meal doesn't have to be expensive to be romantic. One couple I know here in New York has spent their courtship sampling nearly every small restaurant on the West Side. Another couple surprise each other with charming but inexpensive restaurants they've discovered, often restaurants that specialize in Greek, Italian, Indian, Chinese, Thai, or some other ethnic food—where they can dine, romantically, for under twenty dollars.

It is possible to try more expensive restaurants without spending a fortune. "I like to take my girlfriend to the Rainbow Room, Windows on the World, and other fancy restaurants in the sky," says one New Yorker. "I simply ask her to meet me for a drink and we watch the sun set over a glass of wine. Or I suggest that we have breakfast together—preferably after a night together."

Being romantic is a matter of demonstrating how much you care. You don't have to spend a lot on gifts either. Most women are more touched by you standing at the door with a single rose than by two dozen long-stems delivered by a florist. Better yet, surprise her with inventive gifts: fresh strawberries in January, an Italian ice in July, or something special of your own—a book of poetry, for example, that you've read many times.

The most appreciated gifts of all are gifts that demonstrate how well you know *her*—her tastes, her likes and dislikes. If you buy her perfume, buy one you've heard her mention. If she likes classical music, buy a season's subscription to the symphony. If she mentions an interest in learning some new sport, buy her some lessons. "Above all," says one female friend, "never buy her anything that suggests she needs to lose weight or improve her mind."

The biggest complaint among women, however, is that men don't call often enough. One of the best ways to demonstrate that a woman is on your mind is to pick up the receiver from time to time and tell her, especially if you're away or she's away.

If you work in an office, Dr. Machlowitz has some special tips: "Don't have your secretary place your calls to her. Dial the number yourself. And make a point of giving her your private number if you have one. But be sure to give your home number as well, or else she may suspect that you have a wife, a girlfriend, or both stashed away somewhere."

Staging a Romantic Event

Though romance is generally associated with dinner and dancing, it is more a state of mind than anything else. A long walk after a snowstorm is one of the most romantic situations imaginable, providing you're both warmly dressed. Likewise, a walk through the botanical gardens in the spring or through the woods in the fall. Window shopping is romantic, so is browsing through second-hand bookstores or visiting museums. A creative person can make a romantic event take place at the most unexpected moment and can shape it from the most unexpected elements.

I have a friend named Arthur who was moving into a new relationship and a new apartment at the same time.

One day, he invited his new friend, Carol, to see his new apartment. It was still in a state of preparation. The electricity hadn't been turned on yet, and Arthur had to light a few candles. He still hadn't outfitted the kitchen, but he had brought along a bottle of good German wine and two tall wine glasses. He had also installed his stereo, and he was playing some Mozart string quartets when Carol arrived. He apologized about not having any chairs as he motioned her to the quilted sleeping bag he was sleeping on until his furniture arrived.

Arthur joined Carol on the sleeping bag; they finished the bottle of wine with great laughter. The light of the candles cast long shadows over the empty room. They lay down next to each other and made spontaneous, free, and romantic love.

At least it looked that way. Arthur later told me that he'd planned the entire evening carefully. He had put off the delivery of his furniture, borrowed the sleeping bag, and bought the candles all with a view to an unusual seduction.

SIX

Seduction and Arousal

Not long ago, I returned to Washington where I saw my friend Suzanne. Despite the cold, we decided to visit the Rodin exhibition at the National Gallery of Art.

"What are you writing about now?" she asked me with a smile, standing near Rodin's sculpture, *The Kiss*.

"Seduction and arousal," I said, a little reluctantly.

She looked at me askance. "Is that supposed to be a hint?"

"Only if you want it to be," I said.

Then she said something that surprised me. "Which are you going to write about first?"

"What do you mean?"

"Seduction or arousal? Which one are you going to talk about first?"

"Well, they're more or less the same thing, so I thought I'd talk about them together," I said.

The smile disappeared and she suddenly seemed indignant. "What do you mean, 'they're the same thing'? They're not the same thing at all."

I was so surprised, all I could think to say was, "I don't understand. Why are they different?"

Suzanne then began to teach me a lesson that I've since realized is essential to a full understanding of women. "Arousal," she said, "is for dogs. Dogs can get aroused rubbing up and down on someone's leg. Sometimes I think men are the same way. Women get aroused too, because we're animals. But arousal isn't enough, it's not even close. Arousal is nothing without seduction. Seduction is something extra. It's something that happens to the mind. If I'm aroused without being seduced, it's just an inconvenience, like indigestion, or the tickle that makes you sneeze."

Pointing to the marble sculpture in front of us, she added, "I mean, for Rodin, sex was physical, but it was also grand passion."

Whatever you call them, there are really two things that have to happen before a woman is ready to make love. First, she has to *want* it. Her mind (and heart) have to be made ready for it, willing to accept it, emotionally eager for it. That part is what Suzanne would call "seduction," and usually happens out of bed. The second part, maybe the easier part, is physical. She has to be "primed" to make love. Her *body* has to be ready for it, aching for it. That is what Suzanne would call "arousal," and usually happens *in* bed.

I don't think the labels matter. What does matter is that helping a woman reach the stage where she is ready for lovemaking requires attention to both her emotional and her physical needs.

Seduction

What makes a woman *want* to make love? If you asked a hundred women that question, you would get a hundred different lists of requirements. One woman would say, "A tall quiet man, over six feet tall, who is passionately in love with me, a slow ocean cruise, a walk in the moonlight, a pounding surf." Another woman might simply say, "My husband—anytime, anywhere." In the chemistry of the heart, there are no formulas.

There are laws of nature, however. And according to the laws of a woman's nature, there are three things you need to think about if you want to seduce her—if you want to make her *want* to make love.

The Right Person

The most important factor in determining the success of seduction is the person who's doing the seducing. No matter how much attention you lavish on picking the right time and setting the scene, if the woman isn't turned on to you, you're probably wasting your time. Because most women see sex as something far more than merely physical gratification, they're less likely than men to go to bed with someone they don't consider "right." Be self-confident, but also honest. You'll save both of you the awkwardness and embarrassment of an aborted seduction.

The Right Time

For a woman to want to make love, she can't feel pressured by time or other circumstances. That's why seduction has to "fit" into the rest of her life to be successful.

"Even men who are smart sometimes make really stupid mistakes," says an interior decorator in Los Angeles. "Last week I went to dinner with a man I've seen a few times and really like. I started off by telling him that I had to fly to Phoenix early the next morning for a convention, and he *still* spent the whole evening trying to get me in bed. I really wanted to. I kept trying to tell him 'some other night, Dan,' but he thought that was just a line."

Of course, there are women for whom the "right time" is any spare fifteen minutes, who are turned on by the idea of spontaneous sex in unlikely places. But you should be fairly sure of her before suggesting it.

What about her "time of month"? According to Dr. Avodah K. Offit, a sex therapist, women respond differently to sex during their periods. For some, menstrual cramps can decrease sexual interest. For others, sexual excitement can overcome moderate tension or pain.

Some men are put off by the thought of making love to a woman when she is menstruating; others consider it a sign of manhood. Although a man can have little effect on a woman's tension or pain during menstruation, he remains capable of some influence. A woman's reaction to menstruation also depends on her lover's reaction to it. "Men's responses," Offit writes,

"vary from fear of being stained to revelry in a bath of
their lover's rosy flow. Some men insist on towels and
wipe-offs before, during and after; others fingerpaint
their bodies like happy savages in celebration of fertility,
life and love."

The Right Ambiance

Much has been written on creating the right mood
for lovemaking. Cliché though they may seem, I found
the three favorites are candlelight, flowers, and music.
Music can be a particularly powerful aphrodisiac: from
the steady beat of your favorite rock album to the gentle
chords of a Baroque harp concerto, music can set both
the mood and the pace for making love. However, if
you're right for her, if she's right for you, and if the
time is right for both of you, the ambiance is not terribly
important to successful lovemaking.

And I've talked to a great many women who agree.
"The little things are nice, I must admit," says one of
them, "but they're hardly essential. I think too often
they're used as a *substitute* for the real thing in a
relationship. It's sort of like playacting. You know, 'Let's
pretend like we're in love.'"

Although I believe that caring and confiding are
more important in making love to a woman than flowers
and champagne dinners, there are times when a woman
wants to be treated specially. It's at times like these that
ambiance can truly enhance the act of lovemaking.
These are the times to really roll out the red carpet, put
flowers around (or send them to her place), light as
many candles as you can find, put on some soft music,

and, as a friend of mine puts it, "make like a wine commercial."

Just remember, unless you save this kind of staging for special occasions, all the specialness will go out of it. Part of the magic is that it happens only rarely. Of course, the best "special occasions" are the ones you surprise her with for no reason at all.

How do stimulants such as alcohol and drugs affect a woman's level of sexuality? One woman says, "If I'm tense, all I need is a drink or a little grass to put me at ease. Actually, for me, it's the grass that really does it. The great thing about grass is it makes you totally interested in what you're doing. You're totally aware of every nuance of sensation."

The effect of alcohol and drugs depends, primarily, on the amounts taken. If taken too liberally, alcohol and drugs tend to suppress the sex drive. On the other hand, many of the women I've spoken with stated in different ways the same idea: that both alcohol and drugs are very useful in lowering the inhibitions that so often complicate sexual responsiveness.

Will She, or Won't She?

If you're the "right" person and the time and ambiance are, in your opinion at least, also right, how can you be sure that she agrees? How do you know if she wants to make love? Part of seduction is being able to read the signals.

Reading those signals is especially difficult the first time you make love. "All sexual relationships have two phases," a housewife in Boston said to me, "before the first time, and after." Almost all of the men *and* women I have spoken to talk about the first night of sex with a new partner with a combination of excitement and anxiety. Good sex doesn't always happen the first time, but psychologically it can be just wild. For a woman, however, sex is rarely as good the first time as it will be later, after you've made love together many times. But it's still important in setting the tone for later encounters. In fact, how you handle the first time will probably determine whether or not there is a second time.

The first-time hangup men report most often is trying to figure out if their partners really want to have sex. Ironically, one of the first-time problems *women* report most often is not being able to decide if they want to have sex. So it's no wonder the men are confused. How is he supposed to know what she wants if *she* doesn't know what she wants?

A lawyer in Boston confided, "It took me a long time to realize that when a woman says no, sometimes she really means 'Show me how much you want me.' I missed out on an awful lot by believing that first no. A lot of women want to be overwhelmed by a man's desire."

"It's frustrating," says an insurance executive in Hartford. "You start to get hot, she starts to get hot, you're certain that both of you can't wait to get in bed. But just as you think it's a sure thing, a barrier goes up. Sometimes it's what she says, sometimes it's what she does, sometimes it's just a feeling."

HOW TO MAKE LOVE TO A WOMAN

For a woman to enjoy fully the exploration and discovery of the first night in bed, she has to open up, to be completely comfortable, unburdened by reservations or anxieties.

Many women want to become aroused, but don't want to go all the way. What looks like a clear signal that a woman wants to make love may only be a signal that she wants to become aroused. It's a subtle, sometimes wavering line between the two, and one that's very difficult to read.

The most reliable signal is eye contact. The eyes are, indeed, the windows of the soul, and the preoccupation of poets through the centuries with the eyes of lovers is persuasive proof. Dante knew that men and women could say more with their eyes than with their mouths when he said of his love, Beatrice, "Her eyes have shot their arrows into my heart."

Women are as reluctant to answer a direct question like, "Do you want to have sex?" as men are to ask it. "Lovemaking should be like the coda of a Beethoven sonata," says a young female musician in Boston, "the evening should just flow into it seamlessly."

If you want to know how willing she is, the best way to find out is to drop a hint and see how she reacts—with her eyes. The all-time favorite, whether or not it's a first time, is an offer to give her a "back rub." If she's interested, her eyes should shift quickly your way in a look that combines mild rebuke with mischievous interest. You'll recognize the look when you see it. Almost any conversation on any subject, no matter how seemingly innocuous, provides many opportunities for pointed asides and askance glances.

Another "test" is the dance floor. I keep thinking of
what Fred Astaire said about Ginger Rogers: "She was
able to accomplish sex through dancing." I'm also
reminded of what a young doctor in New Haven said to
me about "reading" a woman's sexual desires. "I always
know when my wife feels like making love when we go
dancing," he told me as his stunningly beautiful wife sat
across the room and smiled knowingly. "There's the
weight of her hand on my shoulder, the sudden touch
on my thigh, the slight sigh she gives me when I hold
her closer during the slow numbers."

You can learn a lot more about a woman than her
readiness for lovemaking when you dance with her. A
woman on the dance floor is a kind of pantomine of her
sexual self. I've never known a good dancer who wasn't
a good lover. Interestingly, women say the same thing
about men. "I can watch a man dancing for just a
minute," says one woman, "and know exactly what he's
like in bed: the way he moves his hips, the way he
keeps time to the music, the way he moves around in
his body. It's all there." This is another place where men
can take a lesson.

I like dancing for still another reason. If a woman
doesn't feel in a romantic mood when she steps onto the
dance floor, she probably will by the time she steps off.

Of course, you don't have to go dancing to test a
woman's physical "warmth" toward you. Just see if she
holds "too long" when she hugs you hello, or when she
takes your arm when you cross the street.

"Kisses don't lie," says the old song, and the
women I talked to all seemed to agree. "It's all right
there in the kiss," says a male friend of mine who seems

to have a lot of success with women. "You shouldn't
ever have to ask a question."

Here's a quick primer on kiss-reading, courtesy of
my successful friend. If you kiss her enthusiastically,
does she respond? More important, does she take the
kissing one step further? If you're just giving her a peck,
does she coax your mouth open? Is she the first to use
the tongue? If you use yours, does she follow suit
readily? If the answer to any of these questions is yes,
you can be sure she wants more. How much more is a
question you can answer only by pressing her—gently—
further.

If she does want more, she'll either make her signal
clearer or she'll simply wait until next time. Either way,
you'll get another chance. If she *doesn't* want more, but
you insist on pressing it, she'll either have to turn you
off with a clear rejection or suffer a sexual encounter
that she doesn't really want. That can spell the end of
the relationship. If you force a woman to have sex with
you when she's not ready for it, you may or may not
"get laid," but, in either case, it will take a lot of effort
to persuade her that you're the kind of man she wants
to see again.

If—either at the beginning or at some point along
the way—she shows active restraint, don't press it.
She's sending you a clear message: "I need to know you
better before we go any further. I want to know that
you're the right man." Listen to the message. You're
only asking for embarrassment or resentment if you
ignore it.

If the message is unclear, there's a good reason:
she's uncertain. If that's the case, again, don't press it.

"If there's any doubt about the signals," says my successful friend, "read that as a negative signal." In other words, it's much better to err on the side of restraint than on the side of pursuit.

The safest way is to avoid making love altogether. You don't risk rejection of being told no or the resentment that follows a reluctant yes. As I said before: When in doubt, punt. That goes even if you have your clothes off and are already in bed. "Only a saint can hold back when you've gotten that far," a friend of mine says. "And I'm no saint." It doesn't take a saint, it just takes a little common sense. My unsaintly friend, by the way, doesn't fare very well with women.

Tell her softly that you just want to lie naked with her and feel her skin next to yours. In his bachelor days my friend Ted had a special way of putting anxious lovers at ease. When he knew a woman was nervous, he would tell her that he didn't want *her* attacking *him*, that he'd agree to lie body to body nude with her only if she was willing to restrain herself.

If she was anxious about staying the night Ted offered her an extremely comfortable pair of his Brooks Brothers flannel PJs, tucked her under the covers and kissed her goodnight.

So take your time, don't pressure her. If you're sure she doesn't want to make love, reassure her that, just because you've already gotten your clothes off doesn't mean you expect to consummate the act. There's no such thing as an "obligation" in real lovemaking. Say it with good humor; don't be melodramatic or play the martyr. Remember that what you want is for her to *want* to make love. If she does it out of guilt or a sense of duty, it's not lovemaking at all, it's just "getting your rocks off."

Nothing puts a woman more fully at ease or increases the chances that things will work out better next time than your calm reassurances. Nothing will put her more on edge or make lovemaking *less* likely than pressure—even if it's just psychological pressure. "I don't think there's a woman alive," says a Los Angeles saleswoman, "who hasn't felt trapped sexually. It's almost as if the doors were locked. It can be a real nightmare."

When you restrain the urge to pressure her sexually, you not only save her that kind of anxiety, you "live to love another day." Think of the restraint as a look to the future. You're foregoing hesitant sex today in the hopes that together you'll be able to make love tomorrow.

Here's what a friend of mine, who regularly practices sexual restraint, has to say about it: "Every time I've told a woman I didn't want to make love if she didn't want to, we ended up making love—if not the next time we saw each other, soon afterwards. She knew she meant more to me than a simple orgasm."

Contraception

If a woman is anxious about the first time, it may not be because she doesn't want to make love. It may be something more specific. If you can, you should try to isolate the source of the anxiety: Which female fear is the obstacle? (See chapter 4, "Fears of Flying.")

In many cases, the fear is that of pregnancy. So

begin by asking if she's protected. The tone of your voice is very important. It should be concerned, not demanding or accusatory. "Are you protected?" not, "You are protected, aren't you?"

Even though information about birth control is readily available, many women today are *not* protected. One reason is that the Pill is in medical disrepute and the coil can cause problems. Many women use diaphragms, but you can't expect a woman to always carry one with her when it might be needed. Wearing a diaphragm or carrying one in her bag indicates that she *expects* to have sex, a position of psychological dependency many women would avoid at all costs, even at the cost of no protection.

If she's not protected, you have other options besides complete abstinence. Although intercourse is out, oral sex may not be. A young acquaintance in Vermont told me about his girlfriend from the South who waited until they were in bed to tell him that she wouldn't have intercourse. "It was against her beliefs," he said. "I said okay, it didn't matter—but boy was I amazed when she gave me the best blow job I ever had. Then I did the same for her and she loved it."

A still more responsible option is to provide the contraception yourself. It's the best way for a man to allay the fear of pregnancy because it really demonstrates to the woman that he *cares* as much as she does about the possibility of unwanted pregnancy. Many women are quietly incensed that men are so often cavalier about the risks involved.

The best way to show you care is to be willing to forgo some of your own pleasure in order to protect her.

That usually means using a condom, something that many men resist mightily. A bartender I know in Los Angeles says, "I hate rubbers. Put one on, and you might as well not bother." Even if they don't rob the act of pleasure, they often rob it of passion. "There she is lying there waiting, losing it," says the same man, "while you're fiddling around with your own cock. Forget it."

One way to salvage the situation is to ask her to put the condom on for you. Having her gently unroll the rubber casing along the length of your erect penis can be sexually exciting for both of you. (It can be just as exciting to help her insert a diaphragm, if she has one.) If she knows you're doing it because you care, you can rest assured she won't "lose it" in the time it takes to put one on.

If you decide to use a condom, don't seem eager to use one. Don't have a package of them at your bedside. She may assume that you bought them especially for her visit, or worse, that you keep them handy because you need them so often. Neither is a very flattering—or arousing—assumption.

Arousal

What if you do pick up favorable eye signals or body movements in a woman? If her eyes or anything else "say yes"—making love is the next step. You've won her mind and her heart. It only remains to persuade her body.

If you're alone and able to hold and caress a woman while talking to her, you're probably seducing and arousing her at the same time. But in the normal course of events, many women won't give you a chance to arouse them until you've successfully seduced them. Their bodies follow their hearts—the reverse of many men.

Arousal is a private affair. Many women complain because men try to arouse them sexually in public, by stroking or kissing or some other form of fondling. They see it as teasing more than genuine, caring physical affection, because, as one woman said, "It can't go anywhere." Women tend to be far more physically private than men, and you should keep that difference in mind before you press for anything more than a sociable "peck" in public.

"Arousal," Suzanne told me, "is the art of making a woman ache for love." I can't think of a better description. It begins as soon as your bodies touch and doesn't really end until the instant of orgasm.

Kissing

Many women I know would rather be in bed with a good kisser than with a sexual athlete. In a list of things that really turn women on, knowing how to kiss would rank very high. Women often think of kissing as a special form of communication.

"If the kiss really *says* something, everything else just falls into place," says a student at C.U.N.Y. "If a man takes his time and really enjoys kissing, it makes me feel warm all over and I know the sex is going to be good."

Unfortunately, a lot of men think that kissing is just useless shmaltz unless their mouths are wide open and their tongues are somewhere toward the back of their partner's gullet. For women, kissing is a much more varied and refined art. "French kissing is fine," says one woman, "in its place. But I have to be pretty turned on before I really enjoy it. I like warming up with soft, affectionate kisses. They're much more likely to get me to the point where I want to French kiss." Most of the women I talked to seemed to agree.

So think of kissing in terms of stages. Start with your lips closed. Kiss her softly, warmly. *Tender* is a word that I heard again and again from women: "A tender kiss is a real turn-on." As she becomes sexually aroused, you can begin to kiss more firmly, more wetly, more quickly. Then you can coax her lips apart and test her reaction to your tongue venturing inside her mouth and touching the tip of her tongue. If you withdraw it and hers follows, go a little further the next time. Never push too far too fast; always be aware of her reactions.

Give the woman an opportunity to initiate the kind of kissing *she* likes: let her coax *your* lips apart, let her make the move to the next stage. Part of caring about a woman's feelings is giving her the chance to care about your feelings.

Taking Off Her Clothes

When you undress, the most important thing is to treat her body with appreciation and caring. Since most women are self-conscious about their bodies, you can help put her at ease by keeping the lights low or by lighting candles.

The best approach is to take off her clothes for her. Do it slowly, with deliberate pleasure, before you've begun to remove your own. Appreciate each new part of her body as it is revealed; or, better yet, just kiss it softly and spare the words. When you switch to removing your own clothes, let her reciprocate, but keep your eyes and the focus of your attention on her body.

One man tells me that his favorite approach to disrobing is a variation of the above. He and his girlfriend don't bother to remove their clothes at once; they go to bed clothed, and pet clothed. If you follow his method, disrobing becomes part of foreplay. Instead of breaking the sexual tension to undress, you keep it up, building the tension little by little, piece by piece, as the clothes are removed. Your concentration at this crucial moment in the act of making love is where it should be—on her.

Foreplay

This is the ingredient that women mention most often as "essential" to real lovemaking. Oddly, it's also the ingredient that they complain is most often missing.

The most important point to keep in mind is that what is foreplay for a woman is often direct excitation for a man. If you gently stroke her breast or tongue her ear, that's only a beginning for her. If she does the same to you, an erection is almost instantaneous. And, of course, once you have an erection, you'll have only one thing on your mind—and she'll feel like she has to drop everything else and make it happen.

Timing is the crucial element in foreplay. Because men can be aroused faster and reach orgasm more readily, they often forget that women need more time.

We don't know whether the differences are biological or psychological, but whatever their source, they exist.

So *you* have to take the initiative—especially in the beginning. Give her pleasure for a while without expecting anything specific in return. That way you can give your partner a head start down her longer road to orgasm.

Many of the men I've spoken to seem to think that there's a secret to foreplay—an inside line on arousing a woman without genital contact.

"I like stroking a woman and being tender with her," says a young doctor. "But if I don't have my hand down her pants to see if she's wet, how do I know if she's really excited? It's easy with me. All she has to do is look down and see the bulge. But with her I have to finger her to know, and I can't tell if it's the tenderness or the fingering that's turning her on."

The doctor's dilemma is typical. So many men think that a woman's body really has only two erogenous areas. Nothing could be further from the truth. A woman is a veritable gold mine of sexual sensitivity. There's hardly a square inch of her body that isn't a trigger to sexual arousal if the mood is right and your touch is right.

"I've heard men talk about their penises," says a waitress in a Hartford restaurant, "and that's just the way I feel *all over* when I'm really turned on: just one great big penis. The right touch *anywhere* will set me off."

Petting can involve almost any part of her body; there's hardly a square inch of it that doesn't have the potential to become fully erotic. In my opinion (shared by many men), being a "great lover" means exploring and taking pleasure in *all* of a woman's sexual potential.

Where should you start? Every woman has her favorite place, a place where she's very sensitive and easily aroused. Explore her body and discover her special place. Good candidates are her ears (especially the earlobes), her mouth, her nose, her neck. I've known women who shiver with excitement when you gently massage their hands or their feet.

Try unusual combinations. Instead of simply mouth to mouth, try touching her lips with your finger, or massaging her fingers, one by one, in your mouth. The same thing goes for toes.

Her Breasts

Some areas are more sensitive than others. Breasts, for example. American men are preoccupied by women's breasts. America is practically a cult of breast-worshipers. Yet a common complaint of the women I spoke to is that men don't know how to treat a breast.

"It's such a botch-job, usually," says one woman. "Here they have in their hands the most effective trigger to turn a woman on and what do they do? They squeeze it too hard, bite it, grab it, everything except make it feel good. They're too rough."

Caressing a woman's breasts is an art—a gentle art. Because the breasts' sensitivity can vary from week to week due to hormonal changes in a woman's body, you should always be sensitive to her reactions. There's a fine line between stimulation and pain.

HOW TO MAKE LOVE TO A WOMAN

Begin by caressing the breasts smoothly, brushing lightly over the nipples. Always vary the direction and the weight of the stroke so it doesn't become irritating. The nipples should begin to stiffen. When they do, take one at a time and press it gently into your cupped hand. Now move your hand in a slow, circular motion. The friction will be exquisite and the nipple will be fully erect.

You want to move in stages, each stage more stimulating and more forceful than the last. Never too much too quickly. The next stage is to take the nipple between your lips and alternately lick, suck, and "flutter-tongue" it. All the time you should be kneading the breast itself with increasing firmness (but never too firmly). Some women enjoy it when you use your teeth lightly to "nip" their nipples.

The moment when your face comes to her breast is a special moment. Relish it. Most women find the contact between a man's mouth and their breasts very stimulating. "I think it's one of the key moments in lovemaking," says a housewife. "Somehow, having that man's head between your breasts, his breath on your nipples, his hair brushing against you. *That's* sexy."

The key to arousing a woman is sensitivity. Whether you're kissing, removing clothes, caressing her breasts, or exploring, some women will want to be led, some will want to lead. If you play it right, both of you can be winners in the "courtship game." And you can both share the prize: making love.

SEVEN

Talking

A very attractive woman I know looked at me across the table we were sharing in a fancy restaurant and said in a whisper so loud I'm sure the chef could hear her: "Clint Eastwood is the worst thing that ever happened to my love life." She was so mad, I was afraid she was going to pick up the mousse and fling it at the waiter—but the waiter had heard her and was staying away.

"Jennifer," I said, trying to maintain my calm while everyone in the dining room looked our way, "what's the problem? Is it Dennis?" Dennis was the man she'd been with for a few months. I had introduced the two of them and was happy when they seemed to get along. I almost expected to hear talk of marriage—not movie stars.

Jennifer proceeded to tell me about the havoc Clint Eastwood had wreaked on her sex life with Dennis. Apparently Dennis had learned his "bedroom manner" from Clint Eastwood movies: especially the movies where he was cast in the role of the strong, silent—and sexy—hit man, killer, cowboy, convict, etc., etc.

Jennifer didn't mind the strong part, but the silent part was driving her crazy. "We'll spend a whole evening talking," she told me, "then suddenly, as soon as we start to get it on, he shuts up. And he doesn't say another word until the next morning. He thinks it's sexy if he doesn't say anything. I think it's sick."

The "strong, silent" lover is maybe the best example of how little men know about what women really want. Like Don Juan and Casanova, the strong silent lover is really more the product of men's sexual insecurities than women's fantasies; it's what men *think* women want, not what they really want. "Men just seem to grit their teeth when they get in bed," complains a female associate professor. "They're hell-bent for sex, for the almighty orgasm. It's about as much fun as hunting Moby Dick with Captain Ahab."

Of course, there are a few women who prefer sex unadorned—what one woman called "animalistic lovemaking." Often mistaking silence for passion, they want action, not words. But for most women, talking—verbal communication—is an essential part of good lovemaking.

In fact, words can be the strongest aphrodisiac of all. They're indispensable in the process of seduction and arousal, they can deepen the physical satisfaction of sex itself, and they can foster the postcoital warmth and intimacy that women long for. Given all this versatility and potential, it's amazing that verbal communication is so neglected. One woman, who has traveled extensively, says, "The Irish can talk you into a climax."

Why do American men tend to be quiet? Partly it's

that John Wayne/Gary Cooper/Clint Eastwood image that my friend Jennifer was railing against. But mostly it's their insecurity when it comes to talking: the fear that they'll say something stupid. I think many men have that old saying planted in the back of their minds: "Better to shut up and be thought stupid than to open one's mouth and remove all doubt." Whatever the reasons, many men handicap their lovemaking abilities needlessly by avoiding verbal expressions of love and tenderness.

Before Sex

Obviously, the most appropriate topic for "love-talk" is love. If you're insecure about your own words on the subject, do what suitors did during the Renaissance: borrow appropriate words from the poets. You don't have to make a big deal about it. If there's a poem you like, offer to read it to her; ask if she'll read her favorite to you. If she likes it, make reading a regular thing.

A friend of mine, who has been delightedly married to the same man for fifteen years, still loves it when he reads to her before bed. It's not necessarily poetry. Sometimes it's a novel and he reads a little each night. Sometimes they share the reading.

During Sex

The most important place for communicating—for using a word or two to express your feelings—is in bed. That comes as a surprise to a lot of men who are used to clamming up between the sheets, but almost every

woman I talk to expresses the desire for more
communication during sex.

There's more to talking during sex than just words.
Talking tells a woman that you're interested in her as a
person, not just a vehicle for sexual fulfillment. Women
want to know that men care about their feelings, their
reactions, all during the act of love. When you
encourage a woman to express those feelings, you show
that you care about her; that you're not so focused on
yourself and your pleasure that her reactions are
unimportant.

"A few good words, well placed, can mean the
world," says a New York divorcee in her thirties. "They
add a whole dimension to sex—and they make an
orgasm grow new roots."

The best thing to talk about is her, the things you
like about her. Something personal. Don't talk about
what you're doing or what you're going to do. That
becomes commentary. Tell her what feels good, tell her
how it feels. *Gently*, provide instructions if she asks.
Always encourage, never demand.

If you're not accustomed to words during sex, take
a tip from men in other countries. "The biggest
difference between American men and Italian men,"
reports an Italian fashion designer, "is that the Italians
are much more verbal, much more verbal. For them, sex
is nothing without words, generally strings of
compliments: *'Sei divina.' 'Sei stupenda.' 'Amore mia, sei la
piu bella donna del mondo.'*" In the bright light of day,
these words may sound exaggerated, but in the soft
light of lovemaking, they fall on welcoming ears. An
Italian woman *knows* the compliments are exaggerated,

but she expects to hear them—and she enjoys them.

But there's more to sex-talk than endearments. Words can make lovemaking smoother—it can help you inform each other about what gives pleasure.

Some women are aroused by explicit sexual requests. Others are inhibited by them. You just have to test the waters. "If a man doesn't tell me what he wants me to do, how am I supposed to know?" asks a librarian in Phoenix whose svelte figure and beautiful hair break all the stereotypes about horn-rimmed librarians. "After all, his body is very different from mine. He can't expect me to be a mind reader. You want to know that you're giving him pleasure."

Most of the time, you need to tell a woman what gives you pleasure, and encourage her to do the same for you. There's no reason why you should have to rely only on moans and groans. A moan can't tell you to go faster or to use a different motion, or to do the same thing a little to the left.

"There's something very reassuring about a woman who communicates her pleasure," says one man. "It's like she's in an airport control tower and she's 'talking you in' to a smooth landing. 'I love it when you do that,' she'll say. Or, 'Don't stop.' Or, 'Kiss me there.'" Women enjoy that open communication during lovemaking as much as men.

What about "talking dirty?" Some women hate it, but some women love it, too. Sometimes, the most unlikely women are powerfully aroused by four-letter words: "Suck my cock," "Give it to me," "I want to fuck you."

There's another kind of talk that's almost as bad as

no talk at all. "God knows, you don't want some magpie," says one woman, "someone who, from the moment the first button is unbuttoned, won't shut up."

Another woman related the following story to me: "I went to bed with a newspaper reporter once—what a disaster. We got in bed and right off he started doing a running commentary. You know—'I'm doing this, now you're doing that to me, I feel like this, you must feel like that, now we're gonna do this.' I felt like I was listening to a radio simulcast. He couldn't just let the picture, you know, the visuals, speak for themselves." A woman in Los Angeles said the same thing. "If I wanted a commentary," she said, "I'd ask for a program in advance—or I'd have sex with someone from the Six O'Clock News."

After Sex

Here's where women's needs and men's performance are depressingly far apart. For many women, the period immediately following sex is the crucial part of lovemaking. "It's funny," says one woman, "I'm never really sure I enjoyed it until five or ten minutes after my orgasm. That time makes all the difference. It can make okay sex terrific, or it can make terrific sex dull."

By far the *worst* thing a man can do immediately after sex is roll over and go to sleep without saying anything. Here's a place where talking or saying a few words is *crucial* to a woman's enjoyment or lovemaking. It doesn't really matter what you say. Most women aren't looking for compliments specifically (although if you have one, by all means share it). To a woman, the important things in these first few minutes after sex are acceptance, warmth, intimacy, and caring. She wants to know that what has just happened has some importance.

If you're sleepy, an endearment lets her know you're "there." If you're awake, the intimacy of sex sets the mood for emotional intimacy, for opening up and confiding in each other, talking about recollections from childhood, incidents from the past, problems, jokes, whatever comes to you in that wide-open stream of consciousness after sex.

The one thing you should *not* talk about immediately after sex is problems with the sex. If you want to talk about a sexual topic, wait and bring it up outside the sexual context: during the day, over lunch, driving to a movie—anytime when the subject of sex isn't so threatening. "If there's one thing I hate," says a New Haven woman, "it's instant analysis after sex. I went with someone for a while who regularly gave post-mortems after every time we had sex. He even called them that: 'post-mortems.' He'd say, 'Let's do a post-mortem on that,' and then he'd go on about what we did right and what we did wrong, and I would walk out. It drove me crazy."

"Talk isn't just talk," said a woman I interviewed who's many men's dream of perfection: a former model, now an account executive with a prominent advertising agency. When we started to talk about talking, she waxed almost religious. "Talking is a *lubricant.*

It smoothes the way for everything: seduction, stimulation, foreplay, even fantasy. Conversation makes liking a man easier, seduction-talk makes loving him easier, love-talk makes sex easier. I don't think I could do it without talking to each other, without that feeling I get when a man says something intimate to me."

EIGHT

Technique

You know what really separates the men from the boys? Bed. The boys are the ones who jump in and go straight to work trying to prove something. They want to show you they can get it up, make it last, all that adolescent stuff they get from men's magazines and porno movies. The men are different. They're not trying to prove anything. It all happens so naturally.

—a woman copywriter

So forget performing. Try to forget the image of the playboy, the Casanova, the "lady-killer" that's kept alive by advertisers trying to sell you everything from designer jeans to deodorant soap. In bed, with a woman that you really care about, that image will only make things more difficult and less successful.

For one thing, a woman can tell immediately if you're trying to satisfy *your* needs instead of *her* needs. "I'll tell you honestly," says a New York model, "I hate being in bed with a guy who considers himself a real lady's man. You watch him and it's like he's acting in front of a mirror. He's doing everything to please himself, not to please me. Acrobats, sports fucking, all that's joketime—just showing off."

Of course, "performing" will not only turn the woman off, it's also likely to turn *you* off. If you go into bed thinking that you have to prove something to an unseen audience, you're in real trouble. The woman feels like she's just playing a bit part and you feel like you're on Broadway, opening night, with a house full of critics. That kind of pressure is enough to keep most men flaccid for days.

It isn't just the fact that you're trying to prove something that turns a woman off in bed. Often, it's also *what* you're trying to prove. Most women don't want sex to be "fast, frequent, and furious." Just the opposite. Lovemaking should be slow, special, and sensitive. "Sex—when it's right—is when it all comes together," says one woman, "the attraction, the caring, the touching, the sharing. When it's all there . . . wow!"

Sex—"when it's right"—is the complete act. It's one whole person coming together with another whole person and creating a total bond. It's mutual respect, tenderness, caring, communication, authority, and self-confidence. You should never be happy with sex as mere physical gratification. Women seldom are. It has to be more of a commitment than that, whether for a night or a lifetime. You can only really make love to a woman when both of you are totally involved.

Sex is—partly, at least—a skill. (Actually, I think *art* is a more appropriate term.) It helps to have a mastery of the techniques involved and to practice those techniques. No matter how totally committed you are to a woman, clumsiness in bed can be an obstacle to making love. I've listed below some of the techniques that were mentioned most often by the women I've interviewed.

Masturbation and Oral Sex

"I like intercourse," a female lawyer in San Francisco told me. "But what I really like is when he caresses me with his fingers or with his tongue. It's so pleasurable in so many ways. It helps you relax, it's psychologically reassuring, it helps lubricate the vagina, and it can help focus on the crucial areas—especially the clitoris. So many men think all women care about is how long he keeps his erection during intercourse. If a man really knows how to use his fingers and his tongue, I'd almost be willing to forgo intercourse altogether."

Our culture puts so much emphasis on penetrating that most men aren't aware that penetration is *not* the best way to give a woman an orgasm. Most women require stimulation of the clitoris in order to achieve orgasm, and penetration—regardless of the position—is not the best way to stimulate the clitoris. The fingers and the tongue are far more effective tools: they can be directed more accurately and controlled more fully.

The statistics bear this out. According to a recent study by two clinicians from Michigan, Dana Wilcox and Ruth Hager, only 41.5 percent of women can experience orgasm regularly by penetration alone. *The Hite Report on*

Female Sexuality, a nationwide study compiled by Shere Hite in 1976, was even less optimistic about the effectiveness of penetration. Hite reported that only 30 percent of women can achieve orgasm by penetration alone. Hite also reported that orgasms achieved during genital intercourse are "light," "less pulsing," and "gentler" than orgasms achieved during masturbation, oral intercourse, or some other noncoital method.

Mutual Masturbation

Although most people think of masturbation as something you do to yourself, it is a highly effective tool for satisfying your sexual partner too. Start by touching her entire body: her breasts, nipples, stomach, navel, pelvic bone, inner thighs—everywhere. Only after the body is relaxed do you begin to work your way to the vaginal area. The most sensitive part of the vagina is, of course, the clitoris. But for that very reason you should probably not approach it first. Begin by rubbing the inner lips on either side of the clitoris. You can also try making circular motions around it. A third way to stimulate the clitoris indirectly is to move your fingers inside the inner lips in the area just below the clitoris, so that it tugs at the clitoris itself. All this activity should lubricate the clitoris and prepare it for more direct stimulation.

If there is not sufficient natural lubrication (there are no lubricating glands immediately adjacent to the clitoris; the lubrication must reach the clitoris from within the vagina itself), consider using saliva. The act of taking some saliva from your mouth and pressing it against her clitoris is a turn-on for many women. Or you might use an unscented lotion or jelly. Scented lotions can sting the sensitive tissue. Petroleum jelly is difficult to wash away, but it lasts longer than K-Y® jelly.

Oral Sex

If it's anything women want more of in bed, it's oral sex. In fact, although you may not be aware of it, oral sex is extremely widespread in this country—and women engage in it just as often as men. The 1975 *Redbook* survey found that oral sex is practiced by nine out of ten women under the age of forty and by eight out of ten who are forty or older. Moreover, there was little difference between the number of women who perform fellatio and the number of men who perform cunnilingus. Of all women between twenty and thirty-nine, 91 percent have engaged in oral sex, both active and passive.

"I always have my best orgasms with oral sex," a model friend tells me. "The sensations are so much sharper, much more controlled. It makes me feel as if my lover doesn't just want to screw me—that he really wants to be intimate." It's my experience that almost all women want and expect men to perform cunnilingus—even if they don't want to perform fellatio in return.

The problem is that not very many men know how to perform cunnilingus. More than half of the men I questioned, even those who are extremely active sexually, admitted that cunnilingus made them uncomfortable. One referred to it as a "thankless job—sort of like eating an artichoke."

Even the men who know how to perform cunnilingus well often do it for the wrong reasons.

"Sure, I'll go down on a girl," says a construction worker in Columbus. "I do it to her, then she does it to me." If you feel this way about oral sex, maybe you should reconsider.

Why are some men so reluctant when it comes to oral sex? What do they find so distasteful? "People are always talking about how women don't like to give blow jobs," says a friend. "But I think it's the reverse that's really true: It's the men who have trouble with oral sex, and don't know what to do about it."

Men's basic fear about cunnilingus is that vaginal juices will be unpleasant to smell or taste. And, in fact, just as some men's ejaculate tastes more bitter or more sour than others', some women's juices are stronger than others'. "A woman's taste, her smell can be the ultimate turn-on," a friend in Chicago says. "But if the taste or smell is just slightly too strong, it can turn into a powerful turn-off. It all depends."

Odors are a psychological problem for women as well as men. "I think a lot of women are self-conscious about oral sex," says a young man in New York, "particularly if the man wants to go down on them. They feel somehow that it's dirty, or that it's not really pleasurable for the man, even if the man thinks a woman's sex is the biggest turn-on in the world."

Many women don't equate oral sex with men to oral sex with women. They don't feel it's the same thing. So they don't feel it's fair to ask a man to perform cunnilingus in return for fellatio. Men think it makes women feel uneasy and therefore wait for the woman to ask. But the women don't ask for it—partly because they don't like to initiate this particular sexual activity, and partly because they think men find cunnilingus distasteful. Therefore, it's up to the man to reassure her that he does in fact *want* to perform cunnilingus. That he's doing it for himself as well as for her.

If you've never performed oral sex before, you're missing out on one of the joys of sex. If you're skittish, just take it slowly. You can make sure she's fresh by suggesting a bath together—before you go to bed. Then go one step at a time. For one thing, don't begin with a new lover. You're much better off trying it for the first time with someone you're easy with, and just as important, someone who feels comfortable with having you perform oral sex. "Cunnilingus is where kissing was in the last century," says a professor at Harvard who's a student of modern sexual mores. "Many women resist it unless the partner is right."

Performing oral sex well is not easy for many men. They're trying to give pleasure to a part of a woman's body that they hardly know (comparisons of the clitoris to the penis notwithstanding). "That's virgin territory down there," says a man with a good deal of sexual experience. "No matter how often you've done it, every woman is built different and every woman reacts different. Doing the same thing can send one woman up the wall, make another one uncomfortable, and put a third to sleep."

Because you can't know for sure in advance what will feel good and what won't, you have to pay especially close attention to the woman's reactions. Start out gently and search for the right response. If she's enjoying it, she'll respond. Her breathing will speed up, her hold will tighten, her body will push toward you, encouraging you to continue. As she becomes aroused, the pushing may become more rapid and thrustlike. Be careful not to go too far or to exert too much pressure. Time the movements of your tongue to follow the rhythm of her thrusts.

"Oral sex is like intercourse," says a woman with a New York advertising agency. "You want to harmonize your bodies, harmonize your movements, to intensify that feeling that your bodies are one."

There are some lessons you *can* take from fellatio. For one thing, be gentle. Teeth will hurt her just as much as they hurt you—probably more. For another, vary your activity. Kiss generously, suck gently, and use your tongue inventively: lick, prod, rub.

Start by giving her a few soft kisses along her thighs, moving slowly but steadily toward the genital area. Although the clitoris is your main goal, don't concentrate on it in the beginning as it can be irritating and even painful. Kiss the entire vaginal area, giving special attention to the labia.

Only when the vagina is wet should you approach the clitoris. Be sure to give at least as much attention to the clitoral shaft as to the clitoris itself. If the clitoris continues to be sensitive, approaching it indirectly by licking the clitoral shaft is a way to avoid giving pain in the effort to give pleasure. The friction of a tongue will bring some women to orgasm long before a penis has entered the scene, and many women find it a more intense orgasm.

If you feel nervous about performing cunnilingus for the first time, find the right partner and the right night, then try this trick: Wet your fingers with her vaginal juices, spread them gently across her lips and yours, then kiss. That alone—the combination of the scent and the taste—may soon draw you closer to the source.

Although the tongue has the central role in oral sex, there's no reason not to use your hands too. You can stroke her clitoris while you're kissing her thighs, or massage her thighs while tonguing her clitoris. One woman confided to me that she becomes almost delirious when her lover inserts a few fingers in her vagina, then rubs the wetness across her clitoris, then stimulates her clitoris with his tongue as he inserts his fingers back into her vagina.

Positions

It's high time someone said something in defense of the "missionary position." For too long, people have reviled it as unimaginative, boring, outdated—even sexist. I happen to think its remained the classic position because it remains the most satisfying to men and women alike.

"Missionary position" was originally a term of derision. The natives of Polynesia, who traditionally made love in a squatting position, used it to describe what they considered to be the highly amusing method used by Western missionaries. "It has a bad reputation as being staid, conventional and boring," Dr. Merle Kroop of the New York Hospital-Cornell Medical Center, commented. "[But] it's really a good position with a lot of flexibility. There are some women as well as men who can't reach orgasm in any other position."

There *are* certain disadvantages to the position. First, if a couple restricts intercourse to the missionary position, they have no chance to alternate taking the initiative in making love. If the woman is slight and the man is large, the position can be physically very uncomfortable for the woman. And, of course, the position provides very limited clitoral stimulation.

Despite its disadvantages, however, the missionary position has much to recommend it. Many men prefer the orgasms they have in this position because they can achieve the best control over the depth and pacing of their thrusting. If a couple wants to have a child, the position is particularly conducive to conception. Doctors recommend the missionary position on the ground that it allows the greatest contact of the semen with the cervical mucus. Because the missionary position is traditionally the preferred one and it reinforces accepted sex roles, it is also psychologically very reassuring. Dr. Kroop adds that it is a "very intimate position. There's lots of face-to-face and torso-to-torso contact. It's one of the few positions where couples can really hug, kiss, talk to each other, and feel each other's bodies."

The position actually permits a high degree of penetration, since the woman can regulate the degree of penetration by raising or lowering her legs. "There can be comfortable insertion with the woman's legs down," Dr. Kroop says, "even when a woman is not fully aroused, and the vagina has not yet 'ballooned.' As she gets more excited and the vagina expands, she can raise her knees for deeper penetration."

The Woman on Her Stomach

Don't confuse this with anal intercourse. The woman lies on her stomach and you enter her vagina from behind. Although some women are wild about this position, some don't like it because they can't face you; the visual intimacy is lost. Also, it restricts her caressing during intercourse.

But many women find the pleasures of this position irresistible. For one thing, it permits you to begin with a back rub. More important, you can penetrate farther and more firmly than you can in the missionary position. It also frees your hands during intercourse to stimulate her clitoris. The combination of vigorous pelvic thrusts and gentle fingering sends many women into an ecstasy of repeated orgasms. In making love, being able to give that kind of pleasure compensates for anything you might be missing because she can't reciprocate.

The Woman on Top

Many men and women resist the woman-on-top position because they think it's "unmanly" for the man. In doing so, they're not only showing their ignorance, they're also depriving themselves of a key tool in the art of making caring and varied love. First of all, let's get rid of the male myths surrounding this position.

A man's sexuality doesn't (or shouldn't) depend on anything so arbitrary as who's on top of whom. "Some men get upset when I get on top," says a stewardess in New York. "They think it makes them less masculine, or something. Of all the silly, pig-headed ideas I've ever heard from men on the subject of sex, that's about the silliest."

In fact, for any man who really wants to give a woman pleasure, this position is an essential part of lovemaking. For one thing, the position allows the woman to determine the rhythm of lovemaking, which can often make a vital difference for her. It also opens the vagina wider to allow deeper penetration. It frees your hands to caress her body and, especially, her breasts. Also, because the woman is on top, she can regulate the depth, firmness, and frequency of penetration. That can be not only exciting to a woman, but also reassuring since it puts her in control.

According to Dr. Debora Phillips, another advantage of the woman-on-top position is that it increases both clitoral stimulation during intercourse and the possibilities for complementary manual stimulation of the clitoris. The position is also much more satisfactory when the man weighs considerably more than the woman. The final advantage, however, is psychological. It relieves men of their responsibility. They can lie back and enjoy the act. Some women complain that the woman-on-top position makes them feel ill at ease because their entire body is exposed. You can ease her initial embarrassment simply by closing your eyes the first few times.

If a woman resists taking the superior position, let her know that at least 75 percent of all Americans now turn to the woman-on-top position at least some of the time. A recent study by a Chicago-based sex therapist, Sandra Kahn, notes that a majority of both men *and* women find the woman-on-top position more sexually exciting than the missionary position. She found this to be true despite the fact that most of her respondents assumed that they were in the minority.

The Woman Astride

In the woman-astride position, a variation of the woman-on-top, she *sits*—or *kneels*—with her legs astride your hips. Again, the real plus for the woman is that *she* has control over the degree and depth of your penetration—even more so than in the woman-on-top position.

But there are pleasures in it for you as well. Because the position permits the two of you to look at each other's bodies during intercourse, many women consider it the most visually erotic position. "To sit there and see him stretched out in front of you," says the same stewardess, "to rub his chest or stroke his hair, to dangle my breasts across his face, and all the time feeling him inside me. I'll tell you, it's the best sex I've ever known."

If you make love with the same woman frequently, you'll soon develop your own favorite positions. Your choices will probably be dictated to some extent by the idiosyncrasies of her anatomy—and yours. The nearer the clitoris is to the entrance to the vagina, the more positions you can use; the further away, the more limited you are. The ideal position is the one that accommodates your penis snugly into her vagina and also allows for maximum clitoral stimulation.

A young playwright in New York says, "A man's body fits differently with every woman's body. I had a girlfriend a few years ago and we slept together sort of sidesaddle. Her legs were over me, and I touched her clitoris while I was inside her. It was great. That was how we fit together best. It never felt the same with anybody else. After you have made love a number of times, you'll find a different position, if you're willing to experiment."

Afterplay

"Afterplay" is as much a part of lovemaking as foreplay is a part of arousal. Women unanimously consider the two equally important.

"Most men are good with foreplay," says a female lawyer in Kansas City. "They've learned that they're not supposed to jump right into the act. What most men can't seem to figure out is that they're not supposed to jump right *out*. They're supposed to be supportive when it's over. There's nothing that makes me angrier—or hurts more—than a man who falls into a dead sleep the minute he withdraws."

The exquisite feeling of release that comes with orgasm is followed in many people by a feeling of isolation and loneliness. When that feeling comes, most men are too exhausted to really notice it and their urge is to sleep. Most women, on the other hand, are completely lucid.

Women have a great need to be reassured. They want you to express in gestures and words the same feelings of caring and sharing that you've just expressed in the act of love. If you're really exhausted from the strenuous buildup and release of orgasm, it may take a special effort to give her the attention she so badly needs.

"It makes me furious," says a woman from San Francisco. "I want to ask him, 'How would you like it if I walked out of the room the moment I had an orgasm?' What I love is turning on the bed lamp and cuddling and eating something very sweet like chocolate cake."

"I can't tell you how important it is," says another. "It's what makes the final difference between a physical act, and an act of love."

Making Love to a Virgin

Not every man these days is in the position of making love to a virgin. One man said, "What is a virgin? I never met one!" Men who are in this position should realize that it can be a rare pleasure, but also a pleasure that comes with important responsibilities.

The first time a person makes love—man or woman—is a particularly emotional event. It will probably be a lifelong memory, and will almost certainly color a person's feelings about physical intimacy for years afterward. This is especially true for a woman. The first time may be traumatic for a man, but for a woman, it can be outright painful both psychologically and physically. The man who makes love to her for the first time can put her on the road to a fulfilling sex life, or he can burden her with all sorts of fears and sexual anxieties.

"I've counted it up," says a friend of mine, sheepishly, "and, believe it or not, I've made love to nine virgins. I guess I must be attracted to the situation. A feeling of protectiveness comes over me. I guess I really want to be the one who makes the important event warm and good for her."

If a woman feels anxious about making love with a man for the first time—in particular, if it's the first time with any man—the best way to put her at ease is to make her laugh.

"Before I made love with John for the first time," one woman told me, "I was really scared. I mean, I really liked him, and I was so afraid. I almost didn't want to do it. One night, after a movie, we went back to his place. He had a lot of pillows on his sofa, and we started a pillow fight. Pillow fights aren't something I have every day. Soon we were laughing so hard. From the time we started to kiss and touch each other, it was all so very easy."

If you find yourself making love to a woman her first time, remind yourself how important the occasion is for her. This is one time above all others to put your own sexual interests and needs aside and to concentrate entirely on satisfying her—both physically and emotionally. Unfortunately, for many women, pain will supercede physical satisfaction, but that's no reason why you can't give her the emotional satisfaction she deserves and craves.

Breaking the hymen is the key event. In some parts of Italy today the wedding sheets are still hung from the windows to prove that the young bride's virginity was still intact when the vows were sworn. Of course, some "virgins" have already lost their hymens during sports, masturbation, or gynecological examinations. If not, breaking it can be painful, although the level of pain varies considerably.

Begin with foreplay—as much as possible—in order to relax her body as well as put her mind at ease. Lubrication is also especially important (either oral lubrication or Vaseline® petroleum jelly). Proceed slowly with penetration, accompanied at all times with expressions of love and encouragement. In most cases, when you finally reach the hymen, one quick thrust will hurt less than prolonged pressing.

Immediately reassure her that the pain is over. Tell her, "We have lots of time ahead of us," or "It's going to be better than you dreamed."

Proceed slowly and affectionately. Devote special attention to the time after sex. All women need to be reassured, to be shown how important they are, when lovemaking has come to an end. But nowhere is this truer than when a woman makes total love for the first time.

Above all, a virgin needs reassurance. More so than most women, she needs to feel that the sex came out of caring and affection, not some primal urge. So plan to see her again, as soon as possible after making love for the first time. Wait too long and she may think you've rejected her because she's "compromised" herself. In other words, don't make love to a virgin unless you feel you'll want to make love to her again.

The Big "O"

Nancy divorced her first husband, Ted, a few years after law school and had been seeing an architect, Kevin, for almost a year when I met with her. We hadn't talked very long before she got to the subject of sex. It was obviously on her mind.

"How are things?" I asked her.

"Good. Kevin and I are seeing each other about three times a week. He's so considerate after Ted. It's terrific for my ego."

There was something in the way she said "good" that made the next question inevitable. "How's the sex?" I asked.

She just smiled.

"That good?"

"Pretty good." There was that "good" again.

"Can you elaborate on that?"

"I don't know. It's just much better than it was with Ted."

"You're not really going to leave it at that, are you?"

"To tell you the truth, it makes me mad."

"What does?"

She looked at me hard. "I had my *first* orgasm
about a month ago," she said. "Do you believe it? You
know what that means? I was married to Ted for four
years and I never once had an orgasm. The amazing
thing is that I didn't even know I wasn't having them. It
wasn't until I actually had an orgasm with Kevin that I
realized what an orgasm really felt like—and what I'd
been missing."

"What changed? What makes it different with
Kevin?"

"I don't know. It could be a lot of things. Kevin
makes me feel comfortable. It's so easy with him. With
Ted, I was always angry about something, or on edge. I
was always afraid it wouldn't go well. Even when things
were good, it was like a contest. He was competitive in
everything. I guess he treated sex the same way. I
always felt he was trying to show me how much better
he was at sex. Now I know."

Nancy is not alone. According to *The Hite Report*,
only 52 percent of the sexually active women in the
United States have orgasms on a regular—or
occasional—basis. Think about that for a minute. Not 52
percent of all women, but 52 percent of *sexually active*
women, and that includes orgasms achieved by any
means, oral and manual as well as genital. According to
Dr. Lonnie Garfield Barbach, author of *For Yourself: The
Fulfillment of Female Sexuality,* even those women who do
have orgasms usually have trouble achieving them.

The tragic thing is that, of these many women who

currently are not experiencing the pleasures of orgasm, only a small percentage—the experts aren't entirely sure how small—are clinically frigid. Most are fully *capable* of coming to orgasm.

What this means is that we aren't doing our jobs. A lot of lovemaking is being squandered, or at least monopolized, by men. It means that most of that constant locker-room talk about giving women the "Big O" is just that—talk.

Some men have trouble understanding or sympathizing with this sorry state of affairs. They think women don't need orgasms to enjoy sex. The very same men who can't imagine having sex without achieving orgasm think that women never really miss it. "Coming is what it's all about for a man," says a Colorado rancher, "but women don't come, so they don't care."

Even some doctors—some *male* doctors—have recently argued that people lend too much importance to the female orgasm. While these doctors say that sexual intercourse is important to women, they also say that there is little difference for them between the state of arousal and the orgasm itself, and, therefore, the state of arousal is equally satisfying. These doctors admit that penetration is important to women, but say it's largely for psychological reasons. The very fact that women continue to want penetration, despite the fact that it's not an effective method of achieving orgasm, is offered as further proof that the orgasm itself is not important to them.

A lot of women are quick to disagree with the "experts." One female friend made the point very clearly: "Are you crazy?" she said when I asked the question. "Of course orgasms are important to women. Any woman who doesn't think orgasms are important isn't having them."

Recent studies demonstrate that experiencing orgasm—and experiencing it relatively often—*is* important to most women. In fact, women seem to care more about how often they make love than about how special the lovemaking happens to be. A recent *Cosmopolitan* article, for example, stated that frequency or *quantity* of intercourse may be more important than the *quality* of intercourse. The release of tension provided by orgasm appears to contribute to a satisfying relationship even when each individual act of lovemaking is not treated like a major event.

A 1975 study reported that "for most women, the frequency with which they make love and experience orgasm is related directly to the probability of their reporting a high degree of satisfaction with marital sex."

If ignorance is bliss, then many men live in a constant state of euphoria when it comes to female orgasms. They think a woman is there to maximize a man's enjoyment of sex. Her enjoyment is secondary. "It's real nice when she gets a bang out of it, too," says the same Colorado rancher sympathetically, "it really adds to the pleasure."

In fact, the one with the most potential for pleasure is her, not you. A man's orgasm may come faster and easier, but it's strictly a second-class affair. A man can have one, two, three orgasms during an evening of intercourse. Four sets some sort of record.

A woman can have one orgasm after another after

another after another. Most men, when they hear about the miracle of the multiple orgasms, don't believe it. "I gave my husband a magazine story to read about multiple orgasm," says a Boston housewife, "and he was impotent for a week. He would get in bed and just look at me like I was from Mars. I think it intimidated the hell out of him."

Yet few men—and, for that matter, few women—fully comprehend the nature of the female orgasm. One problem is that you can't really trust a woman's overt signs. Knowing that most men expect and want them to have an orgasm, many women, single and married, fake orgasm. Throughout the ages, women have shown themselves to be great actresses—moaning, sighing, heaving, and throbbing to fake an orgasm at the appropriate time.

Some women themselves don't know whether they're having an orgasm or just a high state of arousal. The Hite study reports that "some women who think they are having orgasms during intercourse probably are not." As proof, Hite quotes some of her respondents' confusing statements on the subject: "There is a deep throbbing inside my vagina when I orgasm," one woman said, for example, "but I have not always been sure whether it was my orgasm or my lover's throbbing."

According to the women I spoke to, however, if a woman isn't sure she's had an orgasm, she definitely hasn't had one—and probably has *never* had one. "Do you know it when you've sneezed?" one woman asked in amazement when I told her the Hite conclusion.

Another woman added, "Of course, as in men,

there are orgasms and there are orgasms. Some are like low tide—just a ripple. Others are like a tidal wave. The last are few and far between—unless you have a great lover."

Generally speaking, a woman's orgasm is comparable to a man's. A male orgasm usually consists of two involuntary responses. The first is a convulsive reaction from the entire body, the second is ejaculation. While these normally take place simultaneously, each can occur without the other. A man can have an involuntary bodily spasm without ejaculation, or ejaculation without the spasm.

In a woman too, an orgasm consists of two parts: an involuntary convulsive reaction similar to a man's spasm, and a contraction of the muscles surrounding the vagina called the pubococcygeal muscle—or the PC muscle. You can feel it contract by putting your finger in the vagina or the anus at the moment of climax.

In fact, all sorts of different things happen to her body between arousal and orgasm. Blood begins to accumulate in the pelvic area; the vagina begins to lubricate; the outer lips, inner lips, and clitoris enlarge (sometimes the breasts also enlarge); the nipples stiffen; and the aureoles—or the darker skin around the nipples—begin to swell.

Then the vagina contracts; breathing speeds up; the pulse increases; blood pressure rises (sometimes the neck, face, shoulders, and breasts appear to flush); muscles in the face, hands, and feet begin to tense up; and finally, the single certain sign, the inner vaginal lips change color from a light pink to a bright red.

It's at this point that orgasm occurs. The muscular tension reaches a peak; the blood pressure, pulse, and rate of breating continue to rise; the tissue engorges even more; the outer third of the vagina contracts rhythmically about every second for a brief time; the uterine muscles, and sometimes the anal sphincter muscle as well, also contract; the blood that has rushed into the pelvic area is released, creating a warm feeling throughout the body.

After orgasm, the swelling of the aureoles recedes, leaving the nipples even more erect; the body perspires slightly; the muscles relax still further; and the uterus and the clitoris return to their precoital resting position. All that remains is perhaps a little pleasant tingling in the clitoris.

Some of these signs of orgasm are difficult to detect. Others are more obvious. I asked many men how they know when a woman has had an orgasm. The difficulty, one said, is that "There are several physical symptoms— her chest becomes flushed, she perspires, her nipples become erect—but not all of the symptoms appear in all women all the time."

A medical intern said, "There's a simple organic method of detecting orgasm in women: I watch her upper chest, around the clavicle. It flushes with pink goose bumps. Of course, there are problems with that. If she's just come from the beach, she could appear flushed for days. And if the lights are out you just can't see."

"It's hard to tell when you're inside," said another man, "but with my fingers, I can tell because the clitoris sort of disappears, and the lips swell up and there are contractions."

"I listen to the pace of her moans, her oohs and aahs," says a lawyer in New York, "if it's very consistent and regular, and then is punctuated by a single variation, she probably didn't really have an orgasm. She was thinking about something that happened at the office yesterday and suddenly remembered she was in bed with you.

"Also, if she gets all gushy, starts saying something like, 'Oh darling, that was wonderful,' and then asks you to come and get it over with, it's pretty certain that her orgasm was based on her desire—her desire to get you out of her as soon as possible."

If you're not sure that your wife or lover is reaching orgasm, you should probably discuss it with her. Just don't raise the subject in bed. In fact, it's probably better not to raise the subject directly. Start a conversation about female orgasm, or orgasms in general, or try to get *her* to raise the subject.

Obviously, the subject is potentially very awkward. One woman said, "Women fake out of compassion for men. To admit you aren't having an orgasm is telling the man that he isn't capable of giving you one. Women think men can't handle the truth. The man has to have the courage to ask the question: Are you having an orgasm?"

How to Help Bring a Woman to Orgasm

What do you do if she doesn't seem to be coming to orgasm? Why are so few women fulfilling their sexual potential? Why are so many men unable to give women full sexual satisfaction? Why is the "Big O" so elusive? And—most important—what can be done if your wife or lover continues to have trouble achieving orgasm?

Nancy's guess at the beginning of this chapter hit the mark. Three decades of psychological studies have confirmed that anxiety and fear, more than any other factors, keep a woman from having an orgasm.

Therefore, it's essential that she be relaxed. If she's uncomfortable or anxious, for any reason, the chances of bringing her to orgasm are very low. That's why most women who have trouble achieving orgasm usually have their first one in an ongoing relationship in which they feel entirely secure. And why most women who have orgasms regularly are sleeping with husbands or lovers in continuing relationships. If a woman is insecure with a man, or if she has any fear—conscious or otherwise—that she may be abandoned, she often can't relax enough to achieve orgasm.

Of course, the best way to help a woman relax is to lavish her with time and affection. One reason most women take so much longer to come to orgasm is that they can't relax without long, consistent physical intimacy. If a woman isn't having orgasms, spend more time with her in bed. Spend as much time as possible— in foreplay *and* in intercourse.

Remember, for most women to come to orgasm, the clitoris, not the vagina, has to be stimulated. In fact, the inner two thirds of the vagina are so insensitive that minor surgery can be performed there without anesthetic. But if most of the vagina is practically insensate, it bears repeating that the clitoris is often much too sensitive. Approach it indirectly at first and always carefully.

Also remember that most women come to orgasm more easily through manual and oral stimulation than through genital stimulation. So concentrate first on stimulating the clitoral shaft with your fingers and your tongue. Especially at first, you can restrict yourselves to the woman-on-top position in order to give her maximum control over the depth and pacing of penetration. It's also important to maintain stimulation as long as possible. Learn to maintain an erection for fifteen or twenty minutes or longer (see chapter 13, "Sexual Therapy"), or else alternate between genital intercourse and manual and oral stroking of the clitoris.

Most important of all: Don't let her bring the stimulation to an end too early. Many women are so conscious of the man's feelings that after ten or twenty minutes, they'll fake an orgasm out of guilt—especially if the man has already come. One man I know was able to bring a woman to orgasm for the first time in her life simply by ignoring her moans and sighs of pleasure and persisting till the real thing happened.

A leading therapist recommends: "Take your time. Relax. Even stop. Talk to her. Play with her. Don't try to be a stud. Appreciate her. Eventually everything will come together." One woman I interviewed said practically the same thing. "What brings me to orgasm? Touching. Kissing. Petting. Licking. It helps if he goes at it a long time. If he's willing to go and stop, and cuddle and go again."

And another: "A willingness to play. If you both climax quickly, great. If you don't, he should touch and tease and kiss until you're so excited you have to climax. But it should be play, not work."

Another woman said: "The most important thing is taking enough time. I sometimes think all men are rushing toward orgasm. I just wish we could spend some time just being intimate. It's partly women's fault. Men are afraid of not satisfying us. I mean, who's putting a gun to whose head? There's a fear of being shown up in bed. It used to be that men would just jump on me and start heaving and hoing. Now they just jump to please me. That's why I usually prefer having sex on weekends or on vacations. I yearn for those periods when we have enough time."

Mary Linda Sara, co-director of the Marital-Sexual Therapy Institute in Fairfax, Virginia, brings up several other points. "A woman requires two things to have satisfactory sex. One, she has to feel completely free of anxiety and, two, she has to be thinking sexual thoughts. Otherwise, orgasm is extremely unlikely. Any kind of fear, any kind of anxiety, can bring an end to the enjoyment of sexuality. If you're making love with a woman and in the back of her mind she's afraid the phone will ring, for example, she'll lose her sexual interest.

"But one of the most prevalent fears is the fear of performance—the fear of *not* performing. The reason most women—and men—lose their ability to perform sexually is because they want so desperately to perform.

"It's like wanting to go to sleep. If you think too much about going to sleep, it's impossible to go to sleep. The same is true of sex. If a woman is preoccupied with having an orgasm, she can't have one—or at least it's a lot harder. It has to come about of its own accord.

Ironically, fear of failure is practically a foolproof formula for failure."

"For a long time," says Dr. Brian C. Campden-Main, a psychiatrist and Ms. Sara's husband and partner, "we thought sex was something you do *to* a woman. Women were brought up to have sex done to them on their wedding night. Then the idea changed. Sex became something a man did *for* a woman. In fact, sex isn't anything you can do *for* anyone," Dr. Campden-Main concluded. "It's something that you can only do for yourself, and a woman can only do for herself. Sex is an activity between two people which they both undertake for themselves *and* for their partner. They can *help* their partner achieve orgasm, but each partner is responsible for his or her own orgasm."

According to *The Hite Report*, "The idea that we really make our own orgasms, even during intercourse, is in direct contradiction to what we've been taught. [But] we do give ourselves orgasms . . . since we must make sure [stimulation] is on target by moving or offering suggestions and by tensing our bodies and getting into whatever position we need." As one woman put it, "You have to go after it."

In other words, the "Big O" is something she has to give herself. What you *can* do for her is help create the right conditions for an orgasm.

If your wife or lover continues to have a difficult time achieving orgasm, convince her that no one *expects* her to have an orgasm. Tell her that, for a set period of time, you won't even expect her to help *you* have an orgasm. Tell her you're glad she can enjoy herself and concentrate on her own physical pleasures.

Think sexy thoughts and tell her about them. Although you can't create a woman's fantasies for her— they're the creation of childhood—you can encourage her to tell you about the fantasies she already has. Let her know that she can confide her fantasies in you by confiding yours in her. The final block to orgasm is in the mind—and a vivid fantasy can sweep that block away.

Single, Multiple, Sequential—and Peritoneal

According to Dr. Avodah K. Offit, the sex therapist, there are three different kinds of female orgasm—single, sequential, and multiple—and they "occur no matter what the site of arousal—no matter where on a woman's body she is stimulated or stimulates herself."

The *single* orgasm is often the first kind of orgasm experienced by a woman. It can be several contractions at varying depths in the vagina, or a single, powerful spasm. Like a male orgasm, the single female orgasm is intense and satisfying. The *multiple* orgasm is a series of single orgasms of varying intensities, one following the other after a period of rest. Shere Hite reports that women experiencing a multiple orgasm can have five or six full orgasms within a matter of minutes. By contrast, the *sequential* orgasm is a series of orgasms, usually not very intense, that follow one another immediately, without any pauses.

Multiple and sequential orgasms have one thing in common: a woman generally develops the capacity for them only with considerable time and experience. Most women are not aware that a different kind of orgasm exists until they experience it for themselves. Experts are not certain what leads a woman to develop the capacity for a multiple or sequential orgasm. Some argue that a new lover, or the same lover using new techniques, can make the difference. Others argue that the woman's own growing emotional and physical sophistication is usually responsible.

Single, multiple, and sequential orgasms do not complete the list. Less well known, somewhat controversial, but more and more talked about is the fourth and final kind of female orgasm: the peritoneal orgasm. This orgasm can give a woman deep, ecstatic pleasure.

It involves the sensitive lining of the abdominal cavity called the peritoneum located deep within the vagina. This "peritoneal" orgasm can be achieved only by the deepest possible penetration; in fact, in most cases, it can be achieved only in the woman-on-top position.

To give a woman this kind of orgasm, avoid elaborate foreplay (especially stimulation of the clitoris). Then, after insertion, apply some pressure to her lower abdomen with your hand.

Stimulating the peritoneum produces in some women an orgasm very different from a clitoral orgasm. It's really more like a male orgasm: it comes rapidly, rises to an intense climax, and happens only once. The peritoneal orgasm isn't easy to achieve. It's what one woman calls "the most elusive 'O' of all."

From Anxiety to Orgasm: Step by Step

What if you've taken the steps outlined above to help bring a woman to orgasm, and she still doesn't have one? Fortunately, sexual therapists have recently developed some remarkably successful methods to help women achieve orgasm. Although serious problems probably require the assistance of a trained therapist, many couples can use these new methods in the privacy of their own bedrooms.

Once you have allayed her feelings of anxiety and done what you can to focus her mind on sexual thoughts, the "cure" will take three steps.

Body Awareness

Women who have trouble with orgasms often aren't really in touch with their bodies. They need to become more aware of its special sensations and responses. Sports can help, but there's also something you can do in the privacy and intimacy of your bedroom. Have her lie down and try to relax as much as possible. Then explore her body with gentle touches, one part of the body after another.

During the first few sessions, avoid touching the breasts or genital area. Doing so will only touch off the expectation of sexual performance. After a few sessions, when you're sure she feels completely relaxed with your touches, you can begin to caress her breasts, and eventually the genital area.

Self-Stimulation

Self-stimulation is the second step. In other words, she should masturbate—preferably with you lying next to her, so that she'll learn to feel comfortable with genital stimulation in the presence of her partner. According to *The Hite Report*, "The percentage of women in this study who never had orgasms was five times higher among women who never masturbated than among the rest of the women."

If she's never masturbated before, now is the time to begin. If she *has* masturbated, she should try using new techniques. If she has always masturbated using her entire hand, for example, she should try stimulating the clitoris alone with one or two fingers. She should continue this until the anxiety goes out of stimulation and she feels entirely comfortable with her body's arousal.

Penetration

The final step is to let *you* stimulate her. Don't try to do too much too soon. Remember, she has to give herself the orgasm. Even when you become directly involved in the therapy, it's still her show.

The idea, however, is still not to bring her—or you—to orgasm. The idea is to make her feel comfortable with penetration. With time and patience and your undemanding support, she'll bring herself to orgasm. If she *doesn't*, it's time to see a professional therapist.

Helping a woman achieve the thundering pleasure of the "Big O" has nothing to do with playing the sexual athlete. It's a slow, supportive, and caring act that requires you to put her pleasure above yours for a while. But when you help her achieve a climax and realize her full capacity for pleasure, you're giving her something enormously important, something that will create a bond between you and bring you an emotional union even more intense than the physical pleasure of sexual release. An orgasm is a gift of love.

TEN

The Spice of Life

Lovemaking is an art. And an important part of that art is variety. There's an old story about a brothel in San Francisco during the Gold Rush where the management "guaranteed" customers a new pleasure every night for a month. Needless to say, the place did a land-office business.

The Gold Rush has come to an end, and according to a lot of women, so has variety in sex. "Everybody has a favorite thing," says a woman in modern-day San Francisco, "and that's all they do. Night in, night out, it's always one or two things. They think it's daring if they avoid the missionary position."

Many women complain that men are boring lovemakers because they aren't willing to try new things, to put novelty or variety back in the bedroom—if it was ever there in the first place.

"It's enough to make you put an ad in the paper, you know, one of those weird underground papers," says an attractive associate in a Houston law firm. "Mine would read, 'Ingenue desperate for ingenious sex.

Submit wildest ideas.' I'll never do it, of course, but it's fun to think about."

Even men who are enthusiastic about trying something new and bizarre are worried about how their sexual partners might react. "You bet I'm curious," confesses a husband in Newton, Massachusetts. "I've fantasized wearing a cock ring for fifteen years. I fantasize it all the time when we have sex. I'd love to try it—and other things. But what's she going to think?"

According to the women I've talked to, she's probably going to think it's terrific. Women tend to be less intimidated by novelty in sex than men, more aware of the role of fantasy. "In the back of my mind, I have a list of things I want to try," says a middle-aged female executive in Hartford with a gleam in her eye, "and as soon as I get the chance . . ."

If you doubt for a moment that women have rich, active fantasy lives, just pick up a copy of Nancy Friday's *My Secret Garden: Women's Sexual Fantasies*. Friday interviewed hundreds of women, asking each of them to describe what they fantasize during intercourse or masturbation. She also published advertisements in various newspapers asking women to send in written descriptions of their most intimate fantasies. Friday received hundreds of remarkably frank responses that revealed that American women have remarkably inventive fantasy lives.

What happens in those fantasy lives? The ingredients are many: rape, bondage, domination, large genitalia, fetishism, bestiality, incest, lesbian encounters, sex with older men, with younger men, with famous actors and famous athletes.

Of course, it's clear that very few of the women would really want their fantasies to come true. A fantasy alive in the imagination complements the physical act and gives it an erotic edge. The woman doesn't really want to be tied up or dominated by some villainous stranger; it's enough to think the fantasy, share her thoughts with her spouse or lover if she can, and perhaps have him handle her with greater authority from time to time.

Why are men afraid to venture too far from the missionary position, or perhaps a little oral sex? Part of it is the same old story: insecurity. The deeper they go into novel kinds of sexual activity, the less secure they feel. "Sure, I've thought about it," says a married man. "I've even fantasized some things I wouldn't want to talk about. But that's a long way from actually doing them. I wouldn't be caught dead doing them."

Another reason men aren't more adventurous in bed is that they're afraid of seeming perverted. They don't think of themselves that way—and they don't want others to think of them that way.

"Sure, there are all sorts of kinky things out there," says a Wall Street lawyer in a three-piece suit, "but they're not the sort of thing people like me do. Can you see me in a leather sling? I can't see my wife in crotchless panties, either."

Ironically, one reason some men avoid the unusual in bed is that they're afraid the women in their lives will like it a little too *much*. These men prefer to think of women they're seriously involved with as virginal—even after years of sex—and restricting the scope of their sexual activity helps maintain that illusion.

Trying to make love with the attitude that sexual

fantasies are somehow wrong is like trying to tie your
shoes with your hands tied behind your back. A man's
fantasies—and a woman's—are as much a part of the
lovemaking act as an erection or an orgasm. In fact,
some experts have concluded that all erections in men
and orgasms in women are fantasy-induced, although
the fantasy may be completely subconscious.

So why suppress the fantasy and limit the fun? Why
avoid new things and risk becoming a boring
lovemaker? Some men feel that a sexual activity is
perverse or unhealthy just because it's unusual or
bizarre. It's not. It's not *what* you do that's perverse, it's
why you do it.

The man who occasionally wants to have his wife
dress up in leather and act the part of a "dominatrix"—
as long as she enjoys playing the part—is doing himself,
his wife, and their relationship a favor. But the man
who can *only* get his rocks off being whipped by a
"dominatrix" figure—no matter who it is—should seek a
therapist.

One of the best ways to enliven any relationship,
new or old, is to explore new sexual possibilities. "We'd
have gotten divorced long ago," says a housewife in
Miami who admits an interest in occasionally covering
her husband's penis with whipped cream, "if we hadn't
been ready to try the unusual. People would be a lot
happier if instead of changing sexual partners, they just
changed what they did with their partners."

Masturbation

Most men think masturbation is a last resort for

lonely nights. In fact, it can be very exciting and very intimate to masturbate together. After all, you're asking her to share one of your most private acts.

A woman in Boston has this to say about masturbation as a part of lovemaking: "Not long ago, I made love for the first time with a man considerably younger than me. After a while, he asked me if I'd mind masturbating a little. He said he'd never seen a woman masturbate and he thought it would be very sexy. I said I'd do it, but only if he'd do the same too. There we were, touching ourselves, without the slightest physical contact. All the intimacy was in the eye contact. I had an orgasm like I could almost see it. And so did he, almost at the same time. He was right. It was *very* sexy."

Taking Pictures

"A lot of women have this model thing in them," says one person interviewed who enjoys taking pictures in bed. "As long as it doesn't interfere with lovemaking, it can be a real kick." If you have a remote-control cord and a little dramatic flair, you can even catch yourselves *in flagrante delicto*—in the act.

Use a Polaroid. That way you're sure the developer won't be able to make a few extra copies, and you'll be able to share the results immediately. Also, consider giving her the pictures when you're through. That way, she'll know for sure that someone won't see them inadvertently.

If you discover that she really enjoys the exhibitionism of it and you own a video and a VTR machine, you might even try making your own X-rated movie. It won't be up to Hollywood standards, but you can play it for yourselves and laugh, or, even better, get yourselves in the mood for a live replay.

Pornography

Many men think that women are turned off by pornography. Even many women are under the impression that women respond more to words than to pictures. A young female writer in New York told me, "Whereas men seem to respond to pictures, women seem to respond better to erotic passages in novels. Why do you think Gothic romances do so well?"

In fact, Kinsey tells us that women are more likely than men to be stimulated sexually by erotic movies and erotic books alike. Men are more likely to *buy* the stuff, however, because most women aren't very comfortable going into X-rated bookshops and cinemas.

The solution is for you to escort her. You'll be surprised how watching *other* people making love can put a sexual woman in the lovemaking mood herself. "I remember walking around Georgetown with a friend," says an aide to a congressman. "I'd been aching to get her in bed, but I wasn't sure *she* wanted it. The signals were confusing.

"We were walking around after a dinner looking for a movie. We walked past this theater and she went over to look at the posters near the ticket office and said, 'This is it.' The movie was *Behind the Green Door*. I was pretty surprised. It seemed like a positive signal! To tell you the truth, the movie was the pits, but what we did back at my place afterwards should have gotten an Oscar."

Sex Toys

Two naked bodies offer so many possibilities for giving and receiving physical and emotional pleasure that you wouldn't think anything else would be necessary. But apparently we aren't even the first society that wanted to improve on nature's best thing. Archaeologists have discovered dildos in ancient Greece, in medieval Japan, and in Africa.

If you think trying novel sex toys will make you weird, you should be aware that 40 percent of the respondents in *Redbook's* survey said they use erotic books, pictures, or movies as a means of becoming sexually stimulated, at least occasionally. And 20 percent have used vibrators, oils, feathers, or other objects in the act of sex.

The most common sex toy is the vibrator. Vibrators come in several varieties. Some fit on the outside of the hand and send their vibrations *through* the hand and fingers. Some are versatile and come with many attachments. The most common variety is the long cylindrical vibrator, what one woman calls "the ultimate dildo for a mechanized society."

Vibrators aren't just substitutes for *real* phalluses when a woman is alone, they're also a common solution to the problem of sustaining intercourse beyond the endurance of most mortal men. In the 1975 *Redbook* survey, 39 percent of all the married women questioned said they took advantage of vibrators during sex.

If you mention the possibility of sex toys and she seems interested, consider taking her to one of the special stores that sell sex toys. The visit itself is often a turn-on to a woman who's always shied away from such emporia. Let her choose for herself from the assortment of ingenious devices: french ticklers (ridged rubber penis sleeves that stimulate a woman to distraction); cock rings (leather, metal, or rubber rings worn snugly around the penis and testicles to heighten sensitivity and prolong erection); and an assortment of leather clothing, belts, and harnesses. You'll have a good laugh if nothing else.

Fantasy can really change people's sex lives. Years ago, I knew a woman named Christina, a buxom blonde from the Midwest who wore tight sweaters—a Lana Turner look-alike. She was in medical school when she fell madly in love with a graduate student from Argentina named Enrico.

One day over coffee, she suddenly became nervous.

"I'm a little embarrassed to say it," she said, "but I'm dying to try bondage and domination."

"Which one?" I asked, trying to restrain my astonishment.

"Bondage. I've always wanted to try it, and I think I should. If I don't, I'll always wish I had. I'm thinking of answering an ad." She showed me the personals section of the newspaper, with an entry circled: *"Good-looking man will provide gentle domination. Will tie up foxy woman and spank her bottom firmly."*

"You've got to be kidding," I said, looking at her in horror. "That would be dangerous."

"Well, maybe a little."

"A little?"

"That's why I wanted to tell you about it. I thought maybe you'd be willing to stay by the phone so I could give you a call if things started to go wrong."

"What good would that do if he ties you up and starts to really hurt you. He's not going to hand you the phone! Have you asked Enrico? Maybe you could try it with him."

"I suggested it to him, and he just laughed. I don't think they have much B and D in Argentina."

"Why don't you give him another try. It's a better idea than letting some maniac tie you up."

Christina did ask Enrico to try it, and, to her surprise, he said yes. To her astonishment (and his, probably), he even liked it.

"It's really improved our relationship," Christina told me some time later. "The sex was beginning to get boring, and this is just what it needed. It's really livened things up. There's only one small problem," she said with a laugh. "Now I want to tie Enrico up."

ELEVEN

Learning from the Pros

During law school, I used to play tennis twice a week with a friend named Roger from Columbus, Ohio. The one thing that always surprised me about him—aside from his great backhand—was how much money he seemed to have. While I was usually strapped for cash, he couldn't seem to spend it fast enough. It was all I could do to make tuition payments. Roger, on the other hand, dressed well, drove a Porsche, and always had a beautiful woman on his arm.

I had no reason to assume he was privately wealthy. As far as I knew, he didn't have a part-time job. It was the great mystery of those days: Where did Roger's money come from?

One night, in the middle of second-year exams, I found out.

It was about two in the morning; we'd been going over cases since the previous morning, and when we finally called it quits, we adjourned to a local bar. Maybe the exam pressure was getting to him, maybe he wanted to titillate or impress me, maybe he just needed to get it off his chest.

Whatever the reason, Roger announced over Scotch on the rocks that he *did* have a part-time job: he was paying his way through law school by selling himself. Roger was a gigolo.

I'd never thought much about gigolos before. I guess I assumed they drove Corvettes, wore gold chains and silk shirts, slicked their hair, and reeked of cheap cologne. I didn't picture them going to law school, or playing tennis—or coming from Columbus, Ohio.

"I never thought gigolos were for real," I said. "You *see* streetwalkers any day of the week but gigolos aren't visible. At least you don't know they're gigolos."

"Well," Roger said, "gigolos aren't really the same as female prostitutes. Women are looking for different things from sex than men are. A man will go out and buy sex for a night. A woman would rather 'keep' a man. She might start paying his bills—taking care of him—and he'll start paying her back with sex. Of course there are gigolos who serve women on a one-time basis but most of them are really just kept men."

When I finally recovered from Roger's announcement, I was consumed with curiosity. How long? How often? How much? But most of all, why?

"I got into the 'profession' sort of by chance," Roger told me. "It started with one of the women partners at the law firm where I worked as a law clerk last summer. About forty-five, honey-color hair. You know, sexy. I've always had a thing for older women.

"We worked late one night and she invited me to

dinner. We drank two bottles of wine; she invited me back to her apartment, one thing led to another and we ended up breaking the basic rule of good office politics. When I got home the next morning, I found three hundred-dollar bills in my pants pocket. Before too long, she had introduced me to a few of her friends. I had a fancier client list than the firm."

Why?

"Obviously, the money's terrific. I mean, even lawyers don't make that much. But the money wouldn't be enough if it didn't make me feel so good. That's right, it makes *me* feel good.

"Most of these women are really unhappy. They're married to stiffs. They're never really satisfied—sexually, I mean. They come to me for that satisfaction: the attention, the affection, you know, all that stuff that they can't find anywhere else. I get off on that."

Roger is still a friend. But his profession has changed. He's now practicing law in Chicago. Last time I talked to him he said, "We just had our third child." Roger's been happily married to the same woman for six years.

Roger's story has stayed with me and led me to wonder: Was there anything to learn from gigolos about making love?

A very successful twenty-five-year-old "callboy" in Chicago told me, "The real trick is to make a woman feel good about herself. When a woman comes to me, I try to make her feel like the most beautiful, the sexiest woman in the world. Some of my clients are getting on in years. They're twenty, thirty, even forty years older than me. That can be pretty awkward, especially in bed. That's the way they want to feel. And the less attractive they are, the more they want to feel that way.

"I start out with something nice and simple, something like 'You smell terrific,' or 'Your nipples are really beautiful.' Pretty soon I can get into something a little heavier. I tell her, 'This really turns me on.' 'You're lovely.' 'I don't want this to stop.' That sort of stuff. It puts her at ease, makes her relax.

"It can be a long night if she stays uptight.

"At first she probably doesn't believe me. She's saying to herself, 'Oh, it's just for the money.' You can see that on her face. But after a while I can usually get her to enjoy herself. Sooner or later, they let themselves believe me because they really want to believe me.

"Sometimes, even I believe me. In fact, most of the time, I can really get into it. You know, it's not just an act any more. Suddenly I *am* attracted to her. I really *like* being with women. I enjoy their company. I just like talking, spending time with them. I bet that's one reason women find me sexy—because I'm really into them, in a lot of ways."

Sean, one of New York City's most sought-after and well-paid professionals works for an agency and specializes in fulfilling women's fantasies.

"You wouldn't believe what some women think about when they're having sex," Sean told me. "The person who's down there (pointing between his legs) is almost never the person who's up here (pointing to his head). A husband or lover is down there, but up here is some college professor they had, some soap opera hero, a famous jock. It's usually the same fantasy over and over, with maybe one or two little things different. It becomes a habit. And she *has* to think about it to get an orgasm."

I asked him for some examples.

"Domination fantasies are big. You know, some guy she saw on the street or the tube that day shows up in her bedroom late at night when she's alone. He rips her clothes off, maybe ties her to the bed, forces her to give him a blow job, call him 'Sir,' makes her beg for more. That's pretty standard.

"A woman may have the exact same fantasy every night for ten years and still be ashamed to say something to her husband about it. She's afraid he wouldn't approve. I don't know, maybe she's right. But if I were her, I'd go ahead and tell him, then ask him to join in the fun. If he's not willing, if he really doesn't approve—well, that's a different problem.

"That's when they call my agency. The agency gets the whole story, details and all, and passes it on to me so I know what to do—what part I'm supposed to play. One of the advantages of working for an agency is that a client isn't afraid of me. She knows I'm not some sort of weirdo. She also knows I won't think *she's* some kind of weirdo, I won't laugh at the wrong time. After all, I do this for a living. She figures I must have seen weirder things in my work—and I usually have.

"I don't think most people really understand what it means to someone to finally live out a fantasy like that, one that's been bugging them every night for thirty years. It's a real kick for me just seeing the pleasure it gives them. Sometimes it's a once-in-a-lifetime thing."

I asked Sean if any fantasy was particularly memorable. He hesitated.

"There was this lady—I guess she was fifty—who had this fantasy about being a college cheerleader. In her fantasy, she waits around after a game for two or three of the players. They come out and surprise her in a dark corner near the field. They're still wearing their grimy, sweaty uniforms.

"She really had the details down. She isn't wearing panties. She lifts her skirt, and one by one they go down on her while she's standing there. Then—she's still got her cheerleader's outfit on, and they're still in their uniforms—she has sex with them, one right after the other. And while she's having intercourse with one of them, she's giving one a blow job and the other a hand job. It's quite a scene.

"The agency really handled that one. They told three of us not to shower during the day, they got us these old football uniforms, and that night in her hotel, we went through the whole fantasy, step by step. It was a blast. I'll bet she's still smiling about it.

"I'm sure that night cost her a bundle. She was probably a little embarrassed at first—jumping around with pom-poms. And we got stares walking through the lobby in football uniforms. But what the hell. That was probably the best night of that woman's life. It was a kick being part of it."

Larry, who lives in a luxurious hotel suite in Atlanta provided by an aging widow of considerable wealth says, "When people figure out that I'm a kept man, they just assume I'm really hung. I mean, sex is my stock in trade, right? I'll let you in on a secret. I'm not. I'm a little under five inches—erect—which means I'm a little under average.

"But a lot of men who are well-endowed aren't good lovers. They don't take their time. Talk about slam-bam. They take it for granted the woman will find everything they do terrific. They don't know a large penis can hurt a woman sometimes, especially if she isn't ready for it.

"Sure, some women like men with big ones. But I think that's an exception, not a rule. But I know for sure, I mean from my own experience, that a small penis can turn a woman on just as much as a big one, if you know how to use it. A man who's small has to make up for it with a lot of foreplay—use your hands, your tongue. A lot of women don't come during intercourse anyway.

"I won't say it's an advantage. When women see me for the first time without my clothes, they're a little disappointed. But they're not for long."

A blond and tanned Los Angeles gigolo who occasionally walks around in the background of shows like *Love Boat* and *Dukes of Hazard* told me that his current lady, a film star of the forties, didn't really want to have sex. "Sex puts her off," he said. "Most of the time, she wants to put her head on my shoulder; she wants me to hold her.

"She knows the sex is there if she wants it. I do whatever she wants. That's been clear from the start. But that seems to be enough—just having it there. I've spent the whole night just holding her—dozing off, waking up and hugging her dozing off. That's not bad. It can make sex better. You know, when you have it. More intense because it isn't automatic. And this is something else a lot of men don't know about. If you wake her up in the middle of the night, after you've both had some sleep, the sex is really hot."

I asked a thirty-two-year-old gigolo in New York, named Jim, if there was anything unusual that his lady friends particularly enjoyed—any "trade secrets."

He thought for a while, then said, "A lot of women like it when I ease my finger up their asses just before they come. It makes them go wild."

Did they ever request anal intercourse?

"Some. About one out of four, maybe."

How did he know when they wanted it?

"It's usually easy. They lift their hips off the bed."

"Aren't they afraid it will hurt?"

"If they've never done it before. But if you do it very gently, it shouldn't hurt too much, especially if she's relaxed. She has to be relaxed. That means you can't do it right away. You can only do it after you've been making love for a while and the juices are flowing. Besides, most women don't mind a *little* pain, as long as there isn't too much."

If a woman wants to have anal sex, Jim begins by wetting the area with saliva. A shower beforehand, he said, can take care of any "esthetic" problems. Then he lubricates the area thoroughly. Although Vaseline petroleum jelly is harder to clean, he prefers it to water-soluble lubricants such as K-Y jelly because they tend to dry out too quickly.

Then Jim massages the anus with one finger, slowly inserting it into the anus. At first the sphincter muscles will tighten involuntarily. You should stop penetrating any farther, he says, until the sphincter has adjusted to your finger. Once the finger has reached the rectum the resistance will lessen dramatically.

Then, to widen the opening gradually, Jim inserts a second finger. Only when the woman is completely relaxed does he lubricate his erect penis with still more jelly and insert it—slowly and carefully at first, ready to withdraw it if the pain becomes too intense. When he's completely inside, he pauses a moment so she can get adjusted. Then he begins thrusting—slowly at first, picking up speed when he's certain she's completely comfortable.

Jim said it's possible to perform anal intercourse in several positions. "The nicest is when she's lying on her back with her legs over your shoulders. That way you can kiss. But if it's her first time, and she's afraid you may hurt her, you can try lying on your back and have her sit on top of you, guiding your penis in herself. In fact, if it's her first time, the easiest position is probably side to side—you know, like two spoons. That seems to cause the least pain."

Jim didn't add—but I will—that you should *always* wash up before reinserting either your finger or your penis in either her vagina or her mouth. Otherwise, serious medical problems can result.

Rick is an in-demand New York gigolo who spent two years as a shortstop on a major league baseball team and still has the manner and physique of a professional athlete. Unlike his colleague Sean, when Rick is sure a woman wants it, he tries to leave the directions up to her. "I just tell her that I'm at her disposal," he says. "What makes me happy is anything that makes her happy.

"At first, some women don't want to give orders. But after a while they get used to it. If they didn't have some desire to control things, they wouldn't be paying for it. The power is a real turn-on for most of them—something they haven't gotten very often in sex. The idea of having me there, ready to do anything they want—or let them do anything to me—they really get off on that. If they want it, I even play the slave role."

What kinds of things do the women ask him to do?

"Just about every woman wants cunnilingus. From what I can tell, there aren't very many men out there who are into oral sex. Women love it, but they don't seem to get it much. I think that's what most women come to me for. They aren't afraid to ask for it."

More of this kind of advice came from a man in Palm Beach, who has the accent and looks of the Latino stars of the fifties and is seen in the most expensive restaurants and clubs with attractive silver-haired women. "You must know when to let her take over," he told me. "A lot of people think I am a big success because I let her lie back and I do everything. It isn't that way at all. It's just the opposite for me. I am a big success because I let her do it to *me*. They like that much better. You have to pick that up quickly, be on your toes. If you push when *she* wants to push, you have a very unhappy lover."

127

"Then you have to be ready if she wants you to take over. I will try it—I'll ask her to let *me* give the orders. I tell her to use her mouth, or to do this or that with her tongue, those kind of things. Believe me, I let her know how much pleasure she gives me. I tell her many many times how good she is to me."

A paid lover in Chicago told me about his specialty: "Massage. That's what I do best. And that's what my women always ask for. I don't mean regular massage— the kind of thing they can get at a beauty salon. I mean a *sexual* massage."

I asked him what the difference was.

"A sexual massage is a massage that leads to the erogenous zones."

Intrigued, I asked for a description.

"Well, I usually use some oil. I like vegetable oil better than baby oil—it isn't absorbed in the skin so quickly—like almond oil, avocado oil, or olive oil. You make them smell better if you add some drops of scent. I use a little of my cologne, so the oil smells like me. Women are big on smells. That way she'll remember me and what I did for her.

"Sometimes, I heat the oil a little. But you've got to be very careful not to heat it too much—you can burn yourself. I always test it by putting a few drops on my wrists before spreading any on her body.

"When you start massaging, don't stop. Even for a minute. If you want to put some more oil on your hands, stay there lying next to her. Put your leg on hers, or your body. Anything so the contact isn't interrupted. Once you've taken your hands off, the spell is broken.

"I work in three stages.

"The first stage is the nonerogenous zones. You know, the back of the neck, the calves, the small of the back.

"Then I turn to the places that aren't really erogenous, but they're pretty close. Like the stomach, the buttocks, the inner 'thighs, the ears, the insides of the elbows, the insides of the knees.

"Finally I turn to the erogenous zones—especially the breasts, the nipples, the vagina. I still think of it as a massage. That's important because that way she can get aroused without getting too aroused—at least not yet anyway."

I asked him to recommend some techniques.

"For the nipples, you should put your two thumbs together in a line, with one nipple in between. Then push the thumbs in opposite directions. Keep on doing that in different positions, around and around the nipple. Believe me, she'll like it.

"With the vagina, I also do something special. If her vagina isn't naturally lubricated, you begin by lubricating your hands. The first thing I do is press the tips of my thumbs against the spot between the vagina and the anus. That, by itself, feels really good.

"Then I push my thumbs in a straight line right up to the inner lips. Then I separate the thumbs, brushing them outward across the outer lips. I bring them back to the inner lips, then back to the spot below the vagina. I repeat that until she's so turned on she can't take it any more. That's when the massage ends and the main act begins."

"If there's anything a woman likes," said a thirty-five-year-old man in Los Angeles who has been kept by a series of women since he was eighteen, "it's staying power. Especially if she can have multiple orgasms—she can only have them if you can keep erect long enough to give them to her, and sometimes that means twenty, thirty minutes or more. Now, it's difficult to stay hard that long without coming. But I've learned to do it.

"The way you do it is you have some multiple orgasms of your own. Most men don't realize coming isn't the same thing as orgasm. Orgasm is that throbbing feeling you get when you come—when you ejaculate—but you don't have to come to have that throbbing feeling. You can get it three, four, five, or even more times before you come. In fact, you can probably get it even more than that, but after three or four, I don't think you get the same pleasure from the orgasm when you finally *do* come.

"So it's great for her, because I can keep it up longer—a lot longer. And it's great for me, because I get a lot more pleasure of my own out of it."

"How does a man achieve these "multiple orgasms?"

"It's a technique that takes a lot of practice. When a man is about to come, the muscles in the pelvis and legs are generally in a state of high tension. If you consciously relax the muscles—let the tension go, the sensations become very intense. You can allow yourself to feel a deep throbbing that approaches orgasm. In fact, it *is* orgasm without ejaculation. Learning to hold back and delay ejaculation without holding back sensations takes some practice. But it has tremendous rewards."

My friend Henry has the final word of advice: "Everything I did was geared to making the woman feel appreciated—that I'd make love to her with or without pay.

"Women used to offer me a tip at the end of the evening. I always refused. I'd say something like, 'No, it was *my* pleasure.' I wanted them to think that there wasn't anyone I would have preferred to spend the night with. After I left, I wanted them to remember it as a real exchange of affection, not just a financial transaction."

If they can do it for *hire*, it should be easy for love.

TWELVE

Keeping Love Alive

Forget everything you've ever heard about the word *tension*. Don't think of it as another word for stress or strain, think of it as a positive force.

In nature, tension refers to the *balance* between two forces. If two planets, for instance, have an equal attraction, there's tension between them. If one planet loses some of its attractive force (gravity), the tension or balance is upset and the two planets either fly apart or crash into each other.

It's no coincidence that men and women act the same way. In any good relationship, there's tension. There's a balance between forces. The man is attracted to the woman, the woman is attracted to the man, and the attractions are more or less equal. If something happens to upset the balance, the relationship is in trouble.

But there's more to tension than just balance. Real tension is two forces coming together and reaching a kind of temporary harmony, a harmony that's stable, but still filled with energy—a good description of the best kind of sexual relationship.

I like to think of this tension in terms of T'ai Chi, an Oriental art that's now becoming popular across the country. In T'ai Chi, there's an exercise you can do with a partner to achieve just the right tension. It's called "push-pull."

You stand facing each other and place both your forearms against your partner's. Then one person begins to push. It's *not* a test of strength. The purpose is to work together with your partner to keep your arms steady and in constant touch, while continuing to push.

You compensate for your partner's push. Do this often enough and you should be able to "sense" the level of pressure, to predict changes in that pressure, and to compensate for them by submitting as they happen. The two of you begin to work as one. The hands may move as the pressure changes, but they remain stable because each of you is compensating for the other's changes. You can even push quite hard, but your partner will anticipate it and compensate by absorbing the force and then pushing back herself.

In "push-pull," a great deal of force, or energy, is exerted through the hands, yet they're stable—in perfect tension. When it's done right, you can almost feel the sparks of energy transmitted between you.

Most of the women I know sense this tension, even if they don't call it that. They know that it's a crucial part of the best relationships. "When I make love," says one woman, "and I mean *real* love, it's like walking a tightrope. I mean we're tightrope-walking together, only we're not afraid of falling. It's a thrill, because we *can* fall—it might not work for some reason—but when it does, it's the best. Some of my best dreams are about being up high. There's a danger of falling—that's the thrill—but I'm not afraid."

Tension is what gives sex and relationships that special thrill. It's that extra something any woman recognizes when she feels it and misses when she doesn't. Tension can come from a lot of things. Like the tightrope walker, some women find that the fear of failure helps create tension. "Fear is right up there," says a friend of mine in New York, "right along with love and sex. It's built into a first date. You don't know what to expect, he doesn't know what to expect. You're both a little scared. If everything works out, that fear is delicious."

But what happens after the first date, or after the first sex? What happens in the middle of a long-term relationship when fear of failure is no longer a real possibility—or at least not enough of a possibility to cause any real tension?

A woman I know who's been happily married for ten years has often complained to me (when we're alone) that her husband Bob is boring in bed. "Our sex is like grocery shopping," she said to me once. "If I'm hungry, the food looks better to me or I buy more, but it's still grocery shopping." That's what can happen if the tension goes out of sex.

Fortunately, fear is only one source of tension in good lovemaking. There are as many others as there are good, loving, sexual relationships—and satisfied women. Best of all, most of the others don't fade as quickly as the first-time fear of failure. Based on the "push-pull" between two whole people, these dynamics keep a long-term relationship alive and growing.

Dominant/Submissive

The old stereotype was that the man was all dominance and the woman all submission. An unbalanced relationship without tension. Now that both partners can take either role, there's an element of uncertainty that is perfect for creating positive tension.

"It's really up in the air," says a teacher in the Boston suburbs. "And that's the way I like it. Everytime we get in bed we have to feel each other out—no, I mean really. That way, anything can happen, and that's exciting. It's been exciting for almost five years now, and I still can't wait to have sex."

Self-Confident/Vulnerable

All people—men and women alike—vacillate between moments of self-confidence and moments of vulnerability. This is a great source of constructive sexual tension. Many women are wildly turned on by self-confident men; but that turn-on quickly fades out if the man isn't capable of vulnerability. "I'll tell you what's sexy," an attractive young female office worker in New York told me confidently, "a man who's so strong he's not afraid to admit he's unsure once in a while."

Many women agree that nothing is more of a turn-off than predictability. A male friend of mine acknowledges as much when he always ends our conversations—especially conversations about sex—with the line "Keep 'em guessing." Anytime there's guessing about what's going to happen next, about whether the man is going to demonstrate his authority or confess his emotional needs, there's sexual tension in the air and good sex in the offing.

Tender/Passionate

Both tenderness and passion have their place in bed, but all one or the other leads to boredom. "Some men are too hyped-up, some men are too wishy-washy," says one woman. "As far as I'm concerned, they're both washouts. The best thing about sex is it's both things at once. Part of me wants to get laid, part wants love. Sometimes I think the only solution is to take two men at once."

A woman shouldn't have to go to that extreme to get satisfaction. A man who is capable of expressing both tenderness and lust will bring the necessary "edge" of excitement to lovemaking all by himself.

Familiar/Unfamiliar

One way to maintain tension in sex is to balance the familiar and the unfamiliar. A woman who likes to play at the edge of uncertainty is a little like the tightrope walker who wants to flirt with failure. There's always a chance of losing something, of making a mistake, of causing pain or displeasure. But that chance is exactly what makes the playing exciting.

"I'm not an experimenter in bed," says a midwestern housewife, "but every once in a while, my husband tries something new, something unexpected.

He's a fox. He does it just often enough so I'm never completely sure he won't surprise me. And they're such sweet surprises, too."

A man who knows how to make love to a woman knows how to use these different sources of sexual tension (and others) the same way he uses different techniques or positions: to make more satisfying, more meaningful love—to make the sparks fly.

For example, a man should be able to sense when a woman wants to play the dominant role and compensate by retreating into submissiveness. But he shouldn't stay there. Like the T'ai Chi partner, he should always be applying pressure to dominate—not so much pressure that he discourages her efforts to dominate, but enough to maintain the tension, the uncertainty about what will happen next.

By the same token, a man should know when to respond to a woman's self-confidence with vulnerability, and when to "answer" tenderness with passion. "One of the things that makes sex so good is that it's so complicated," says a pretty account executive at a midwestern retailer. "There's so much going on at one time. There are so many possibilities. I think of it like those acts in the circus where the man keeps fifteen plates spinning at one time. Good sex is like that."

It helps to be aware of the role of tension in lovemaking. It's so easy to fall into patterns, into routine ways of doing things and responding to situations. Many of the married women I've talked to say this is their main problem in sex. "It's all so predictable," laments a New Jersey housewife. "I know when he's going to moan. I know what he's going to say, the way he grits his teeth."

"I'm just as bad as he is," admits a married woman in New York City. "Every time it's the same thing. He does this, then I do that, then he does this. Sometimes I feel like I'm in a long-running Broadway show."

If a man can learn to understand the idea of creative tension in a relationship—whether or not it's in bed—then he's mastered a whole new way of bringing energy to a relationship. But to achieve creative tension really requires the full participation of his partner. The man must anticipate and promote the woman's active involvement in the act of making love. It's not something that a man can just bring home one day and impose on a relationship. The learning process, like T'ai Chi's "push-pull" has to be mutual.

THIRTEEN

Sexual Therapy

Many men with severe problems are afraid to visit a sex therapist. No matter how much their relationships are suffering, they're still reluctant to seek professional help. "I've only had two real problems in my family," says a Connecticut housewife, "getting my son to have his wisdom teeth out and getting my husband to see a sex therapist."

Women aren't the only ones who find convincing a man to see a therapist like pulling teeth. The therapists themselves complain that men are always dragged unwillingly into their offices. "In any couple I see," says a well-known New York sex therapist, "there's always one person who's really the moving force, the person whose idea it was to come to me in the first place. Nine times out of ten—no, ninety-nine out of a hundred times—it's the woman."

Why are men so reluctant? Partly, it's a macho hang-up. One of the great lines from John Wayne movies is when the Duke reprimands some younger man for saying "I'm sorry." "Don't apologize, son," he growls. "It's a sign of weakness." For all too many men, agreeing to go to a sex therapist is like saying, "I'm sorry we're having sexual difficulties." It's a sign of weakness.

Men tend to be so much more sensitive to sexual criticism that they're willing to do anything to avoid it. They're afraid of having to wear a big red "I" on their coats that will brand them forever as impotent, or "PE" for the dreaded premature ejaculator. In their hearts they're so afraid these things are true—and irreversible—that they can't bear the thought of confirmation by an expert.

Even the suggestion by a wife or friend that they could be helped can be mistaken for a serious rejection.

"When my wife said something to me about sex therapy, I went through the ceiling," said one of the few men who would even discuss the issue with me. "I thought she was trying in a very subtle way to tell me she wanted a divorce. I couldn't sleep for a week and the idea of sex turned me off completely. I thought, 'Now I need therapy.' And so she won."

Don't assume from men's reluctance to seek professional advice for sexual problems that they don't need it. Masters and Johnson estimate that about half of the men and women in America are involved in a relationship that has some sexual problem or another. And judging from the women I've interviewed, that estimate might be conservative.

"I don't want to tell you how many men I've slept with," says a pretty red-headed computer analyst in her twenties, "but I would guess three or four had serious problems—and I mean serious."

To learn more about sexual problems and sexual therapy, I went to a prominent Chicago psychologist who specializes in sexual therapy. I wanted to relay what he told me so that the men reading this book can get a better understanding of what a sex therapist can do, and perhaps even effect a home cure.

Why Do Men Have Sexual Problems?

For men as well as women, fear and anxiety are the main culprits. "This is an elementary lesson," says the Chicago psychologist and therapist. "If you're worried about performing, it's much more difficult to get it up and keep it up. If you're having trouble with an erection, your anxiety breaks the meter and you haven't got a chance in hell of getting an erection.

"The problem is, you can't get an erection until you regain your self-confidence, and you can't regain your self-confidence until you get an erection. The therapist's job is to halt this downward spiral before it gets entirely out of control."

Occasional sexual problems can often be solved, however, simply with the help of a concerned and caring sexual partner. "There are all sorts of 'home cures' for minor sexual problems," says my therapist, who's also a psychologist, "assuming, of course, that you've got the right sexual partner."

By the "right sexual partner," he means someone who's willing to place a higher priority on your sexual needs—and solving them—than on her immediate sexual needs, someone with whom lovemaking is a caring experience, someone who cares more about making love than having sex.

What Can You Do About Impotence?

"I'm about ready to give up sex altogether," she began dramatically. "I've been to bed with seven men in four months—*seven*—and the sex hasn't worked out a single time. I feel like such a failure. I see a man several times, we like each other, we go to bed, and something goes wrong. He can't get it up, he comes too soon, it's always something.

"My worst experience was with Jon," she said, "this guy from the office. He was terrific. Sensitive, smart, a good sense of humor. The first time we went to his place we got in bed and petted for a while and it was great, but then nothing happened. I began to feel pretty strange. I mean he was lying against me and there was no erection, nothing.

"Then he told me that he had to give himself a hand job to get an erection. That threw me. For fifteen minutes he tried. That was bad enough, but he wasn't even having any success. It was really depressing. After a while, he suggested that he take me home. I haven't seen him since. It's a shame, but I really don't know how to deal with the problems."

I asked the therapist what he would have told Nancy if she had come to him.

"The problem is that many women, especially young women, blame themselves for erection problems.

' "But as women grow older, they generally become more understanding. Most women like a man who's vulnerable, honest, and needy on occasion. They also like being assured that a man wants to have sex to express his love, not just for sexual release. If Jon had been honest with her, she probably would have given him just what he needed: lovemaking without the pressure of sexual performance."

I asked several women how they'd react to such an unusual request. One woman, a friend in Boston, told me that one man, a man she found very sexually attractive, actually came to her with the request. He didn't apologize about the problem, she said. He just told her about it in a matter-of-fact way. Instead of being turned off, she was delighted that he had enough confidence in her to share his problems so openly. "It was wonderful," she said, "so honest and intimate.

"It was a challenge. It appealed to the savior complex in me. It excited me to think I might be the first woman who could bring him to orgasm. I also found it rather freeing—it put me in control. Of course, sometimes it was frustrating as hell. It took me three months before he felt comfortable enough to get a real, satisfying erection. But it was rewarding. Our relationship eventually broke up and I'm still close to him. Women who take impotence as a sign of rejection are missing a lot."

I asked the therapist in Chicago how he would suggest Jon deal with his problem.

"He's got to realize that he can't wish an erection into being. A penis won't perform on demand. Only sexual excitement can make a man stiff. The more he worries about an erection, the more that worry will smother the sexual excitement, and the less likely an erection becomes. By far the best cure for impotence is to go to bed consciously rejecting the possibility of having an erection and engaging in intercourse.

"He could do anything else he wants. Kissing, petting, oral sex. But he *shouldn't* try to become erect. If he begins to stiffen after a few evenings, he shouldn't try to do anything with it. He shouldn't try to hurry it along. When he begins to stiffen as a regular thing— which he will, unless his problem is medical—he can begin to penetrate the vagina.

"I would recommend that he let *her* insert his penis so he doesn't get distracted by the mechanics of the process. He should be focusing on the pleasure. Once it's in, he should thrust it in and out slowly. He shouldn't worry if he begins to lose the erection. It will come back—if not that night, then the next night. Also, I'd tell him not to worry about an orgasm—either his or hers. That's only more pressure, and pressure's the last thing he needs.

"If he does these things, and he really conquers the worry, it will happen. Eventually, he'll have an orgasm—there won't be anything he can do to prevent it. And once he gets his first orgasm, he's over the mental block. From then on, he shouldn't have any problem."

What Can You Do About Premature Ejaculation?

Many men—perhaps a majority—ejaculate long before they've brought a woman to orgasm. The result is that many women—maybe a majority—are dissatisfied with their sex lives.

"Premature ejaculation," of course, is a relative term. An ejaculation is only premature because it comes before a woman's orgasm. There's no published schedule, it's just a matter of timing your ejaculation to maximize a woman's pleasure. The problem is that most women take longer to reach orgasm than men. It might take them twenty minutes, or even longer.

Of course, you can continue to massage her clitoris long after you've come yourself. But sex will be far more pleasurable for both of you if you learn to maintain an erection as long as possible. It *can* be done. In fact, in Indian Tantric sexual practices, the ultimate sexual achievement for a man is the ability to perform intercourse for more than an hour and *never* ejaculate.

What can a therapist do about premature ejaculation?

"There are any number of *bad* ways to prevent premature ejaculation," said my therapist. "Since the cause of the problem is up here [in your mind], many cures try to turn your mind off sex while turning your body on. They try to get you to think about some unrelated object, or to distract yourself with pain— usually biting or pinching.

"The problem with both these approaches is precisely that they do detract from your concentration. I remember the wife of one of my male patients saying something like, 'I don't care if his penis is still in my vagina. Who cares about his penis when his heart and mind are watching some baseball game? It's *him* I want, not just his genitals.' I must have said it to a hundred patients. In making love, concentration is more important than penetration."

What are the "good" ways to prevent premature ejaculation?

"As with any therapy, the first and most important thing is a cooperative, caring partner. The procedure is known as the 'squeeze technique.' It's complicated, but reasonably foolproof—as these things go.

"If a man is about to ejaculate, he can usually stop it by pressing his thumb against the frenum—that's the sensitive underside of the penis where the glans, or head, meets the shaft. You need one or two fingers on the other side for leverage, but all you have to do is just squeeze a little, not too hard. It only takes a few seconds.

"You can do it yourself, or you can show your partner how to do it. Of course, if it's your partner, you have to let her know when to apply the pressure—how to feel with her fingers the throbbing that indicates imminent orgasm. Avoid intercourse at first; ask her to stimulate you orally or manually. After she's learned to time her squeezes pretty carefully, she can mount you from the top and insert your penis in her vagina, with her fingers grasping the base of the penis.

"This first stage is just penetration, not intercourse. Let her control the motions, the in and out, to relieve you of all responsibility. Man-on-top positions are out. When you're about to ejaculate, *she* should withdraw your penis and apply the squeeze. After a while, you'll be able to hold an erection much longer without ejaculating."

A few men's sexual problems are physiological in nature. They *always* have trouble getting an erection. Anyone who has persistent sexual problems should investigate the possibility that the problem is really in your body, not your mind. Diabetes, endocrine diseases, lesions of the central nervous system, too little arterial blood, and an overuse of drugs have all been isolated as causes of impotence.

It bears repeating, however, that the proportion of sexual problems that are caused entirely by body misfunctions is very small. For every man who has a physiological problem leading to impotence or premature ejaculation, there are hundreds who suffer from occasional impotence or premature ejaculation for psychological reasons: too many worries at the office, too much to drink, too much anxiety about sexual performance. There's a list of causes as long as the list of victims.

Serious, persistent sexual problems—even of a psychological nature—require the help of a professional.

FOURTEEN

A Living Fire

Not long ago, my friend Suzanne made another visit to New York. When I met her at the airport, I marveled at how beautiful she is. Even through the crowd, I could see the sparkle, the life, in those large eyes. I suddenly had the feeling we would become lovers.

Driving into the city, I told her the book was nearly finished but I was having trouble with the ending. It was somehow incomplete—something vital was missing. She offered to come back to my apartment and have a look.

We took off our coats, I poured two glasses of brandy, and she followed me to the desk. It was covered with squeezed up balls of paper.

"What is it that you want to say?" she asked.

I thought about it for a minute. "I'm still trying to convey something of the mystery that takes place when two people love each other. You know—that serene, intense happiness you feel when you make physical love. For many people, I think the sexual experience is a spiritual experience—maybe the only one they ever really have."

"Hmmmm," she said, leafing through the pile of sex books I had accumulated in researching the book. "What do you mean exactly?"

"Well," I said, "when you touch a woman you love, I think you make a link that's much more than just physical. It's as if your fingers are rooted in her body. There's an immediate connection. It's like energy passing from you into her, and it gives every movement, every sensation, every pleasure, an extra dimension.

"I think that's what every woman longs for. That certain something is what makes sex into love and men into lovers.

"And I think every man is capable of communicating that certain something to the woman he loves: of making her feel she's part of him and that he's part of her. You don't need any special talents. You certainly don't need special looks. All that's needed is the courage to take emotional risks, to open yourself up to the ecstasy of two people becoming one.

"If you focus all of your attention and your affection on her, the contact between your bodies will be alive with sexual electricity. You'll share the rarest of all intimacies.

"If she responds the same way, your bodies will flow into one another at the points where they touch— and at the eyes. The two of you will be joined in the kind of perfect, mystical—almost spiritual—union that's the essence of making love."

"I think I know what you're getting at," she said softly. "I've got just the thing for you. Why don't you quote from D. H. Lawrence? I know you have *Women in Love* because I borrowed it from you once. Let me show you a passage from it. Where are your novels?" I led her to the bookshelf and after a few minutes of searching I pulled the well-worn volume from its place. She sat down next to me on the couch and read for a while. Finally, she turned to me, her hand on my arm, saying, "This is it—my favorite passage:

She traced with her hands the line of his loins and thighs, at the back, and a living fire ran through her, from him, darkly. It was a dark flood of electric passion she released from him, drew into herself. She had established a rich new circuit, a new current of passional electric energy, between the two of them, released from the darkest poles of the body and established in perfect circuit. It was a dark fire of electricity that rushed from him to her, and flooded them both with rich peace, satisfaction.

'My love,' she cried, lifting her face to him, her eyes, her mouth open in transport.

'My love,' he answered, bending and kissing her, always kissing her.''